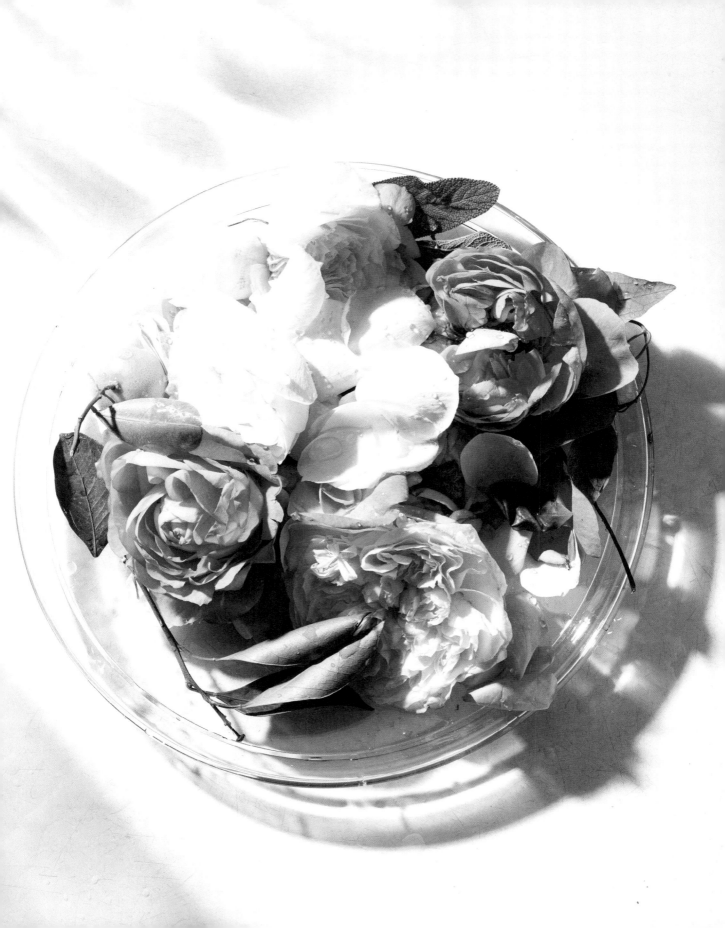

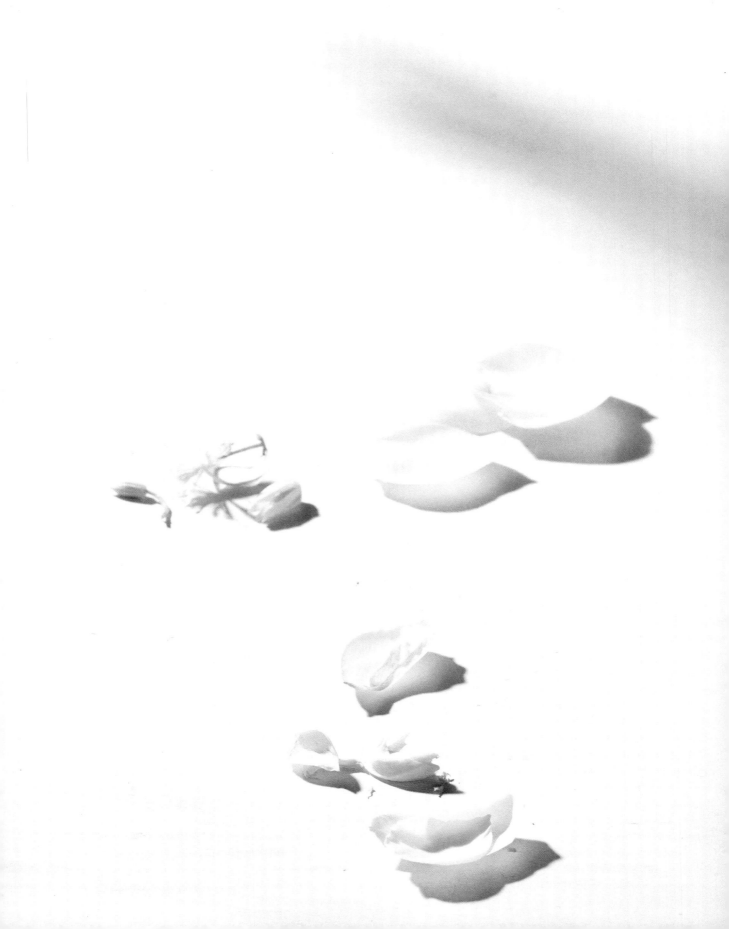

The
Naturopathica Effect

*A Holistic Approach
to Skin Care*

Barbara Close

NATUROPATHICA®

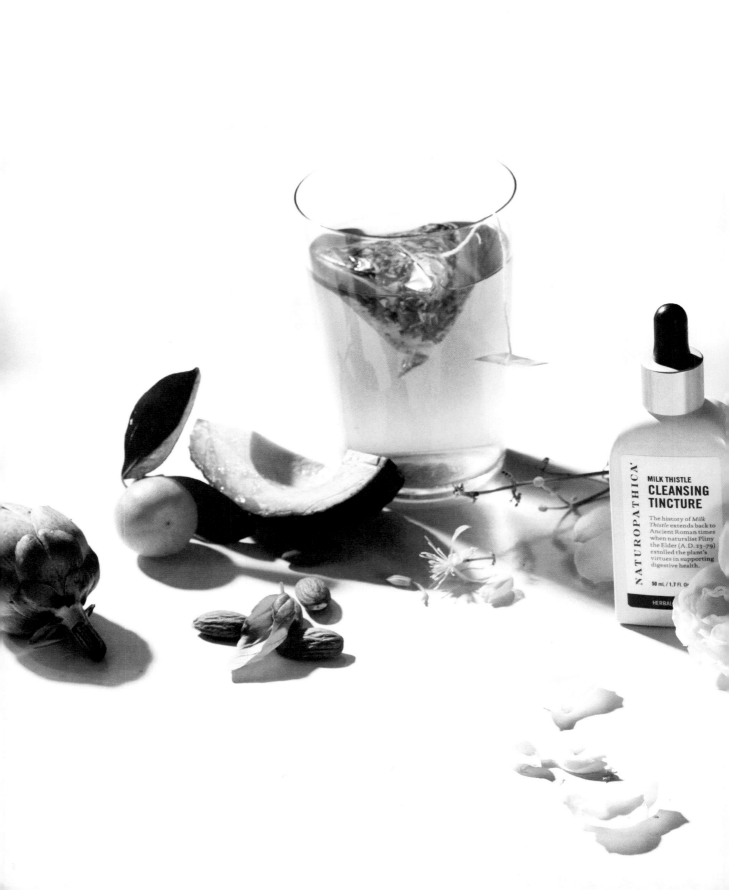

Contents

Foreword

The hottest beauty buzzwords in America today—clean ingredients, holistic self-care rituals, botanically-derived ingredients, heck, even beauty foods—didn't sprout from the ground and land on your Instagram feed last year. They were seeds planted and watered more than a decade ago by women like Barbara Close, Naturopathica's prescient and pioneering founder, and a practicing herbalist and aromatherapist.

Trends come and go, but the early aughts were a time when the beauty world was smitten with cosmeceuticals, ingredients born in the lab, and endorsed by a celebrity doctor. I was a beauty director then, writing about the science of skin care, often through a spa lens for the long-ago shuttered Luxury *SpaFinder* Magazine. This is when Barbara, a Hamptons spa owner for 10 years who'd trained dozens of healers at top spas to use her botanically-driven products, landed on my radar.

Her way of talking about beauty was totally different. Instead of megaphoning the virtues of lab-coat innovations (even though her skin care line also used amino acid peptides, fruit acids, and potent vitamins and she very well could have), Barbara woke me up to the performance of plants. Their healing potential according to several schools of plant medicine, their biocompatibility with the skin, their power to affect stress, sleep, digestion, and pretty much everything I personally worried about.

Barbara's brilliance wasn't that she'd solved my skin care goals, it was that she spotlighted the factors that effed up skin in the first place. "My goal was to create a path to healthy beauty that takes into consideration the world we live in," she said. And that's a holistic take that goes way deeper than even an excellent moisturizer can.

There were only a few American brands in fall 2006 that were built on the notion that every ingredient in your beauty product should be non-toxic and actually do something for your skin. Naturopathica was the most well-known, but it was still stocked alongside the dermatologist brands, even though it was telling a very different story. I featured Barbara in a landmark beauty feature called *The Purists: Five Entrepreneurs at the Forefront of the Natural Beauty Revolution,* where her ethos came through. In the piece, she also wore a frilled Etro button-down that we both remember as the farthest thing from "hippy" ever.

I wasn't an easily swayed journalist. But a kind of stealthy logic started to take hold for me—that traditional beauty brands and approaches were imitating what botanicals effectively had the lock on for centuries (until the early 20th century when beauty was industrialized and commercialized).

Barbara explained how plant stems, roots, oils, extracts, and leaves were the foundation of her apothecary-style products, and I began to lose my enchantment for the miracles of marketing and promises problem-solved in test-tubes. "Contains vitamin C" or "includes natural antioxidants" were bragging rights of brands whose products barely included a whisper of plants in them. And yet they were selling their science.

In our teched-up lives, where stress, leaky gut, and inflammation issues are as common as your phone battery dying, beauty has very little to do with skin care at all. In fact, if you're Barbara, and you see the world through a lens of health, you do what you can to get out of its way. You consider the toolbox of the herbal apothecary, and how plant remedies, sippable elixirs, aromatherapy, water cures, massage treatments, meditation, and, well, lots of things will benefit your skin, but sometimes don't even require making direct contact with it.

That's the approach of the gorgeous Naturopathica location in the Chelsea neighborhood of Manhattan. It's become a destination for holistic skin care, where your healing protocol may include drops of **Inspire Aromatic Alchemy, Vitality Tea,** and **Milk Thistle Cleansing Tincture,** alongside use of the **Manuka Honey Cleansing Balm** and **Plant Stem Cell Booster Serum.**

A beauty healing journey, like any healing process, is a necessarily self-led one. Hence the update to this gorgeous book that Barbara wrote 13 years ago. The tried-and-true basics of *The Naturopathica Effect* are presented with up-to-the moment intel for today's clean beauty customer: How to incorporate the right herbs into your diet and life, beauty food recipes, and lifestyle tips that all lead your skin to its birthright—a healthy, glowing state.

The essence of what more people seek from beauty brands today is an ally in the skin's healing process, and transparency around ingredient sourcing, whether topical or ingestible, to back that up. And while many are scrambling to tell this story, Naturopathica's has been long documented. "When the rest of the industry comes around," I wrote back in 2006, "they'll find the Purists like Barbara are already there."

—Melisse Gelula, Co-Founder, Well+Good

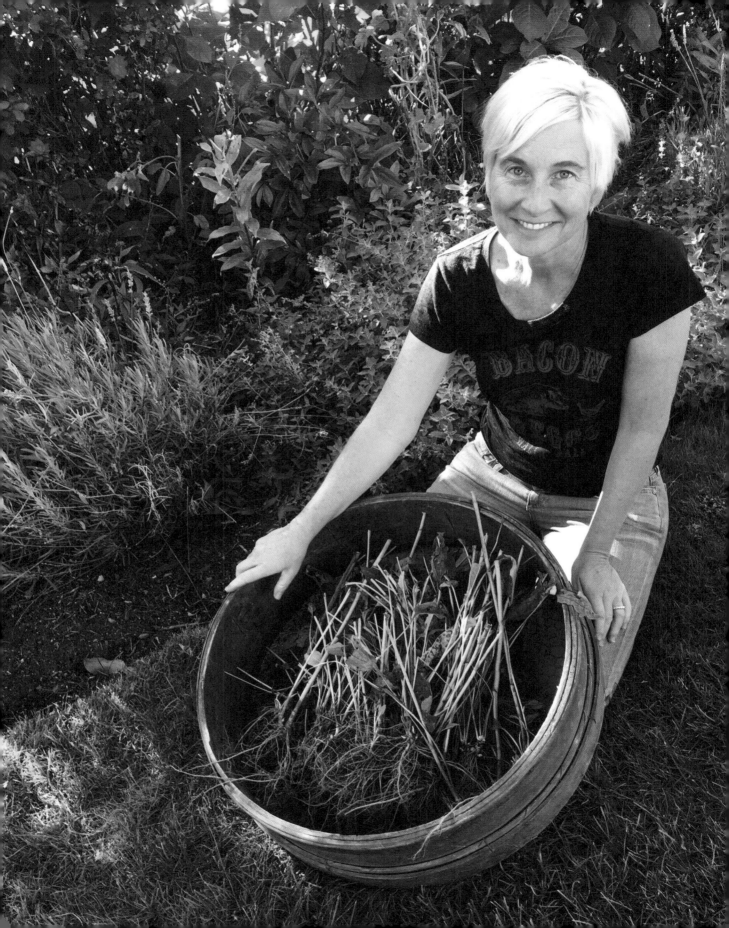

Introduction

Of all the gardens of my youth, the one I hold most dear belonged to my grandfather, the proud owner of hundreds of acres of rolling green hills and rust-colored soil in Virginia. I recall the myriad scents I gulped in as a child running across that rambling farmstead—waftings of wild carrot, the smell of newly turned soil on rapeseed fields, the aroma of dried leaves, blackberries, rose, rhubarb, and honeysuckle, and the one fragrance I remember most by far: that of the Madonna lily, whose sweet scent of decay in the warm afternoon sun haunts me to this day.

Scent is a bewitching and magical muse. It holds the ability to conjure long-forgotten moments of delight from your past and induce feelings of peace, comfort, and joy in your present. The transformative power of scent to shift our consciousness and our emotional response to everyday stress is a pretty remarkable feat when you think about it. And yet this is only one example of the infinite therapeutic properties found in a holistic approach to improving and maintaining your health and well-being.

I am often asked how I became interested in holistic health and natural skin care. I don't think I realized it until after she was gone, but my great Aunt Eleanor, an ex-pat who lived outside of Paris, offered me my first vision of the benefits of natural health. Viewed by many as a bit of an eccentric, she eschewed prescription drugs, preferring to visit the *herboristerie*, where they would prepare a *verveine* tea to assist with sleep, or recommend a chamomile-and-yarrow salve, to help with dry skin. Europe has a strong ancestral knowledge of herbal medicine which, sadly, we have lost in America with the rise of the pharmaceutical industry. My aunt loved to visit mineral spas regularly to "take the waters," and I enjoyed soaking with her in the thermal pools and mud baths. Above all, Aunt Eleanor thought that food was the best medicine, primarily fresh fruits and vegetables along with protein like chicken or fish and an avoidance of all processed foods.

Years later, after graduating from massage school and apprenticing with herbalists in Santa Fe, New Mexico, my formative years with my aunt were put to intensive use when my mother was diagnosed with lung cancer. I witnessed firsthand the inability of Western allopathic medicine to offer anything in the way of palliative care to help her cope with her illness. I was awakened to the healing potential of lemon-balm tea to ease her anxiety, homemade calendula salve to help with radiation burns and dry skin, peppermint inhalations to quell nausea, and weekly aromatherapy massages to soothe her muscle pains and stave off headaches. As I witnessed the effectiveness of these traditional healing arts, I became determined to create a place where other people could learn about self-care rituals to improve and empower their own well-being. Three years later, in 1995, my vision for Naturopathica was realized when we opened our first door in East Hampton, New York.

Scent is a bewitching and magical muse. It holds the ability to conjure long-forgotten moments of delight from your past and induce feelings of peace, comfort, and joy in your present.

CORE PRINCIPLES OF NATUROPATHIC MEDICINE

The Healing Power of Nature
This principle is grounded in the belief that the body has an innate ability to heal itself.

Do No Harm
Holistic skin care never uses toxic or irritating raw materials that would be detrimental to the health of the individual.

Treat the Cause
The root causative factors have to be addressed to treat an imbalance.

Holistic Approach
Skin disturbances usually have multiple origins stemming from and/or affecting mind, body, and spirit, each of which must be addressed.

Prevention
A good skin care regimen focuses on preventing imbalances instead of treating symptoms.

From the beginning, my goal at Naturopathica has been to educate people about natural health and beauty in new and exciting but accessible ways. I define beauty not as a pampering or indulgent experience, or a quest to achieve an artificial, idealized form of beauty, but as an expression of living an authentic, healthy, and vibrant life that celebrates one's own unique beauty and spirit. This type of beauty is rooted in wellness, in achieving one's full potential. The problem with much of the culture of beauty today is that it relies on quick fixes like Botox and plastic surgery or the latest hyped-up miracle cream, and so remains indeed only skin deep. Feeling beautiful is no longer about "beauty secrets"—being confident in our own skin comes from making connections between our lifestyle and how we look and feel. This type of beauty is not about shoring up on the outside and looking for "hope in a jar." It is about being at home on the inside—a genuine organic beauty.

This is the essence of holistic skin care, and the foundation of this book. Holistic skin care encourages you to be an active participant in your own skin health by supporting the body's own natural healing processes, and is based on the core principles of naturopathic medicine (left).

The Naturopathica Effect: A Holistic Approach to Skin Care is designed to show you how to practice holistic skin care that nurtures a radiant inner beauty, providing all the inspiration, resources, and practical advice that you will need—and striving to educate and assist you in using nutritional medicine, aromatherapy, herbal remedies, massage, bath-water cures, and mind-body techniques to transform how you look and feel.

The first chapter, "The Skin You're In: A User's Manual," focuses on the fundamentals of skin but moves beyond the usual skin typing (normal/dry/oily) to help you better understand your complexion. This section launches the holistic approach to skin health and explores how problems such as acne, rosacea, or sensitive skin are usually reflections of imbalances on a deeper level, such as oxidative stress, blood-sugar imbalances, hormonal changes, nutritional deficiencies, or chronic inflammation. In Chapter 1 we will also explore exciting new research on the skin microbiome, a highly complex ecosystem that provides a home for billions of bacteria on the surface of the skin and plays a significant role in your skin health.

Developing an understanding of your "skin personality" readily leads to a more comprehensive approach to creating personal skin care routines—your beauty basics. Chapter 2, "Customized Beauty Rituals for Your Skin Personality," explains why skin-typing is an insufficient diagnostic tool for determining why you may be experiencing skin imbalances. Instead, I use skin personalities, which give a complete view of your skin health by looking at your diet, stress level, hormone balance, and skin care habits. In this chapter, you'll learn how to identify your skin personality and discover the remedies and rituals, that will help you care for your skin.

The power of plant materials to improve the health of your skin is explored in Chapter 3, "Pure Ingredients, Pure Results: Skin Care Recipes." This section cuts through the hype and marketing of the beauty industry to give you the bottom line on harmful ingredients in skin care products. You'll discover the sad truth that many common over-the-counter cosmetic ingredients are potentially irritating and toxic, and learn how to read cosmetics labels. Next, the active benefits of essential oils, pure vegetal oils, plant enzymes, and botanical extracts are explained, so you can know what to look for when you shop for healthy skin care products. This chapter goes further by providing techniques for blending aromatherapy ingredients and recipes for even the most difficult skin care problems, so you can create your own natural products at home.

We are all too familiar with the old adage, "You are what you eat." Succumbing to convenience foods that are empty of nutrients makes us look and feel bad, and yet often, with the circumstances and pace of our lives, may seem inevitable. Chapter 4, "The Beauty Kitchen," will help guide and inspire (or reinspire) you to eat well, and offers simple strategies that make good, healthy foods just as convenient. One of the most important and exciting research trends right now is the study of how imbalances in the gut, or digestive system, can lead to chronic inflammation and create a host of disorders such as asthma, allergies, and even sensitive skin. People with sensitive skin, including acne, may experience flare-ups as a result of a shift in gut health. This chapter will help you recognize and understand the key signs of toxic overload, and provides guidance for better nutritional choices with shopping lists and recipes that promote gut health and enhance healthy skin. By eating delicious, nutritionally rich foods, your skin will be nourished internally, thereby slowing down the body's natural aging process.

The fifth and final chapter, "That Which Adapts Thrives," explains how to adopt the staple therapies of natural healing—bath-water cures, massage, aromatherapy, herbal medicine, and meditation, to name a few. My Aunt Eleanor had flawless skin, which she attributed not only to the benefits of natural health but also to Dr. Erno Laszlo, whose elaborate rituals such as his famed "double cleanse," complete with thirty splashes of hot water performed twice daily, left me mesmerized. To this day, well-being rituals are the essence of Naturopathica's holistic health-care prescription, as these simple self-care techniques have the ability to inspire and empower us to live and feel better every day.

The essence of beauty lies within: when we feel our best, we look our best. Ultimately, beauty is an attitude, an approach to living. In *The Naturopathica Effect: A Holistic Approach to Skin Care*, I tried to assemble a thorough, enlightening and entertaining owner's manual for your skin, and I hope it will help make looking after yourself simpler and more pleasurable throughout every stage of your life.

Chapter 1

The Skin You're In

A User's Manual

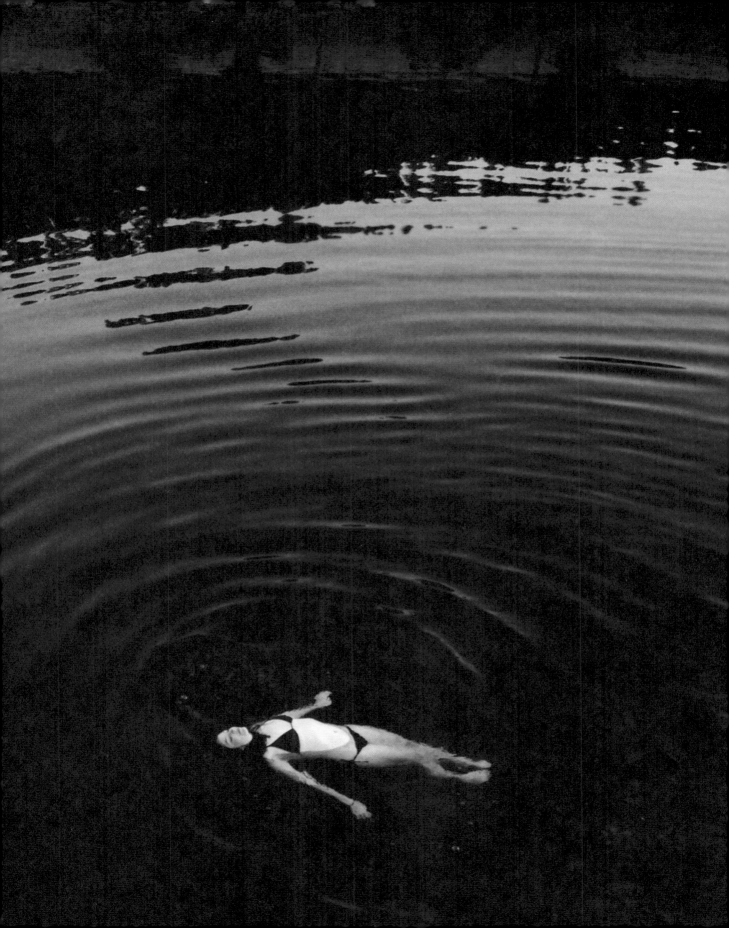

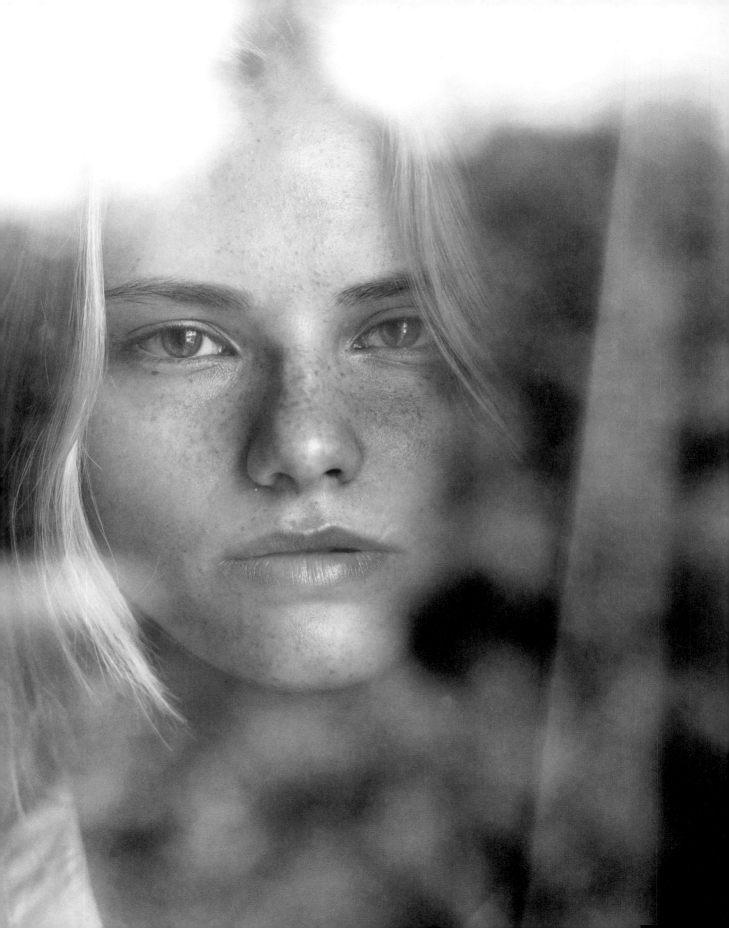

We all seek remedies that will unravel the mysteries of our skin's constantly evolving landscape and provide the key to guaranteed radiance. But as much as I want clear, radiant skin—I have to believe in the process by which it is achieved. If there is one thing I cannot face in a beauty regimen, it is a heavy dose of hype.

What I am looking for is true skin care: an attainable, gentle, results-driven practice that produces honest beauty and allows me to enjoy the ritual, while at the same time, assuring me that I am not damaging my skin or compromising my health. And so, along the same lines, I don't believe this should entail endless hours of protocol or require dozens of excessively expensive products.

This school of thought begins with an understanding that your skin is much more than just a cellophane-like wrapper around all the important stuff. It is in itself a vital organ that has the often thankless job of blocking out the bad elements—bacteria and viruses, for example—and is also always working to protect and nourish the body through processes such as temperature regulation, excretion of water and waste materials, and absorption of vitamin D from ultraviolet sunlight.

None of this usually comes to mind, of course, when you wake up one morning and find your chin mapped with a constellation of blemishes. The human body is a giant communications system, and nowhere is this more apparent than in the skin, as it is the perfect reflection of what is going on inside the body. The Chinese use the skin as a diagnostic tool because it is connected to all the systems of the body. When our digestion, blood-sugar level, nervous system, or hormones are out of balance, our skin will tell the story.

Every Face Tells a Story

Have you ever wondered why symptoms such as redness, bumps, dryness, changes in pigmentation, or blemishes suddenly emerge on your skin, only to disappear as if they had a mind of their own? Or why it is that some of us seem to grow old gracefully—that is, smoothly (literally)—while others of us watch the skin around our eyes take on crow's feet and our forehead and cheeks start to resemble the Great Barrier Reef? The simple answer is that the skin is constantly changing, and flawless skin is a combination of good genes, lifestyle, and beauty regimen. But the truth is more complex—symptoms are messengers for change. The real cause of imperfect skin comprises five main factors that often overlap: oxidative damage, blood-sugar issues, nutritional deficiencies, hormone imbalances, and inflammation. These factors all define your unique and evolving skin personality.

Oxidative damage refers to free-radical theory. Free radicals are oxygen molecules that bear free electrons. They are highly reactive and can weaken proteins when the body becomes vulnerable. As a result, nutrients are

The human body is a giant communications system, and nowhere is this more apparent than in the skin, as it is the perfect reflection of what is going on inside the body.

locked out and wastes kept in, so cells grow rigid, leading to wrinkled skin. With overexposure to external environmental aggressors, such as the sun and pollution, as well as internal factors, such as a poor diet or chronic lack of proper hydration, symptoms like irritated skin or premature wrinkles may result.

Blood sugar can also play an important role in the aging process. When high levels of glucose are present, the glucose can bind to the skin's collagen and elastin, creating a process called *glycation*. The end products are called *advanced glycation end products,* or AGEs; these create irreversible cross-links between adjacent proteins and contribute to a loss of elasticity to the skin, typically resulting in cracked or red skin as well as wrinkles. Maintaining an intake of low-glycemic (low-sugar-forming) foods goes a long way towards preventing this inflammatory response. (This phenomenon will be explored in more detail in Chapter 3.)

Nutritional deficiencies most often occur in individuals who have poor diets, consume excessive amounts of alcohol, and/or have digestive issues. While conventional medicine often downplays or even discounts the connection between skin health and nutrition, there is strong evidence to support the influence of our food choices on the health of our skin. Vitamins and minerals—as supplements or, preferably, through your diet—can play an important role in addressing skin imbalances. For example, several studies have indicated that zinc can help reduce acne symptoms, as well as other skin disorders such as the small white-and-red bumps called *keratosis pilaris* that some of us find on the backs of our arms. (We'll also discuss how dietary sources of vitamins and minerals can help support healthy skin in Chapter 4.)

Hormones are the chemical messengers in our bodies that travel in the bloodstream. Their role is to communicate with organs and tissues, and it only takes a small amount of any one of them to cause significant changes in the body. Many hormones play a role in the skin, from cortisol, which influences inflammation and sebum production to melatonin, which affects our sleep to sex hormones such as testosterone and estrogen, which can promote undesirable effects like acne while performing their main functions. Hormone fluctuations can wreak havoc upon the skin, but fortunately, there are treatments and lifestyle changes that can help keep them in balance.

While by now many of us are aware that **inflammation** is a causative factor in illnesses ranging from heart disease to Alzheimer's to cancer, the range of things it throws out of whack in the body is huge and a matter of intense ongoing study.

WHAT ARE THE CAUSES OF INFLAMMATION?

Externally, when your skin is exposed to irritations like UV light, polluted air, or averse chemicals such as the ingredients in some skin care products, your body initiates an inflammatory response and may exhibit symptoms such as redness, swelling, and heat. Internally, inflammation occurs when your body engages the immune system to attack a foreign body—anything from a mosquito bite to an ulcer in the lining of your stomach.

You may be surprised to learn that the gastrointestinal (GI) tract is the seat of our immune system, as almost 75 percent of our immune cells live there. Our gut, specifically the small intestine, is home to countless bacteria—both good bacteria, such as *Lactobacillus* and *Bifidobacteria*, which protect us from deadly pathogens, as well as harmful bacteria, like yeasts and parasites. According to the National Institute of Health, up to 70 million people suffer from digestive disorders, but scientists do not know why digestive imbalances are on the rise.[1]

One unifying theory is that these imbalances might be driven by increased permeability of the gut (aka "leaky gut syndrome"; see sidebar), which promotes chronic systemic inflammation throughout the body as our immune system responds to the influx of microorganisms.[2]

This systemic inflammation weakens natural immunity and inhibits the body's reactions to everyday challenges, such as preventing sun damage or acne. Here's the bottom line: If your body is busy engaging in a battle to fight inflammation, it cannot focus on the necessary daily processes it needs to perform for your skin, things like making collagen and elastin.

INFLAMMATION & PREMATURE AGING

Chronic inflammation causes premature aging of the skin because it promotes free radicals, highly reactive oxygen molecules that damage cell membranes by stealing electrons through a process called *oxidation*. At the same time, your body releases three key enzymes—hyaluronidase, elastase, and collagenase—which break down hyaluronic acid, elastin, and collagen, the main building blocks of the skin.

One key to protecting the health of your skin is to avoid skin irritants found in many conventional skin care products (see page 51). As an herbalist and product formulator, I wanted to use only ingredients that support the skin's health to fight inflammation. As an esthetician, I wanted to go further and added clean cosmeceuticals to our formulas—active ingredients such as plant stem cells and fruit enzymes that produce change in the skin without irritation.

Whether you choose to use my products or follow the recipes in this book to make your own skin care products, my goal is to help you understand the importance of controlling inflammation.

A GUT FEELING

Factors that may contribute to increased permeability of the gut include:

American Diets High-sugar foods, processed foods, and carbohydrate-heavy diets trigger the release of cytokines, signaling molecules made by cells that regulate inflammation.

Chemicals NSAIDS (a category of anti-inflammatory and pain-reducing drugs including aspirin and ibuprofen), pesticides, cosmetic irritants, mercury exposure, and other everyday chemical agents can trigger an inflammatory response in the skin and body.

Stress Stress triggers the release of cortisol (see "The Stress-Less Step," page 27), which mobilizes blood sugar, in turn promoting inflammation.

HOLISTIC BEAUTY BASICS: 10 EASY STEPS

The essence of holistic skin care is simplicity. Striving for good skin does not mean you need to keep your medicine cabinet packed with a vast assortment of bottles and jars containing ingredients with seven syllables in their names. What your skin really wants is a dose of common sense and TLC, not product overload and complicated beauty regimens. For most of us, this might be as simple as using the correct cleanser or applying a vitamin-rich avocado oil at night.

Step 1: Cleanse, Don't Strip

Cleansing, the most important step in your beauty ritual, lays the proper foundation for correcting or fortifying your skin. The purpose of cleansing is to remove dirt and excess oil, both of which can block pores and lead to breakouts. Skin cleansers are typically made up of three main ingredients: a surfactant, or wetting agent, to reduce surface tension on the skin; oil to help dissolve grease; and water to wash away dirt and grime. In order to clean the skin, a cleanser has to break down the hydrolipid barrier of the skin, the delicate layer of surface lipids made up of oil and water.

Unfortunately, this is not as easy as it sounds. Your gut is not the only place brimming with beneficial bacteria; your skin also has its own microbiome, a collection of millions of tiny organisms on the surface of the skin. Using cleansers loaded with antimicrobial ingredients or harsh surfactants wipes out the good bacteria.

A good skin cleanser will not strip the hydrolipid layer, which would take away the naturally good oils of the skin along with the grime. Nor will it alter the slight level of acidity that is normally found in the skin and acts as a barrier to limit bacterial overgrowth. This is why you should never use soap, even handmade soap, on your face. Its alkalinity will upset the pH balance, cause irritation, and leave the skin feeling taut.

After you cleanse, you'll want to tone your skin. The role of a toner in the cleansing regimen is to correct the pH balance of the skin. Contrary to popular belief, toners cannot help to "tone" your pores, because your pores do not open and close. However, toners can deliver beneficial ingredients, such as those in essential oils, to the skin. For example, some toners, called floral waters or hydrolats, are natural by-products of the distillation of essential oils. Hydrolats contain microscopic particles of the plant material suspended in water. Sprayed regularly onto the skin, these tiny particles behave similarly to homeopathic medicines to help the skin stay balanced.

A CROSS SECTION OF THE SKIN

Human skin has its own ecosystem that depends on a complex series of chemical processes. The cycle begins with building up plump new layers of cells rich with collagen, the main structural protein. These cells flatten out as they move towards the surface, and they are discarded when they reach the uppermost layer of skin, the *stratum corneum* (epidermis), every 14 to 28 days.

Imagine the *stratum corneum* as a brick wall. The bricks are composed of these dried-out cells held together by lipids, which are like cement. The *stratum corneum* is often referred to as the "skin barrier," and protecting the strength of the skin barrier is an important key to healthy skin.

Below this layer lies the dermis, home to two critical types of connective tissue, collagen and elastin. These two tissues are responsible for the strength and elasticity of the skin.

Nerve endings, hair follicles, and sweat glands are all embedded in the dermis. A network of thin blood vessels, called capillaries, helps move nutrients to the uppermost layer of the dermis and remove by-products of cellular waste.

The subcutaneous layer, the deepest layer of the skin, provides support for veins and internal organs and is made up of fat cells that help the body retain heat. Here, new skin cells are formed from nutrients carried by the capillaries.

Your skin is a vibrant organ that interacts with both internal and external forces on a daily basis as it seeks to maintain balance. A commonly held view, that the skin is basically a membrane best left to topical treatments, is extremely simplistic. Understanding the actual depths of your skin reveals the importance of being an active participant in your overall health and taking a holistic approach to nurturing well-being and preventing premature aging.

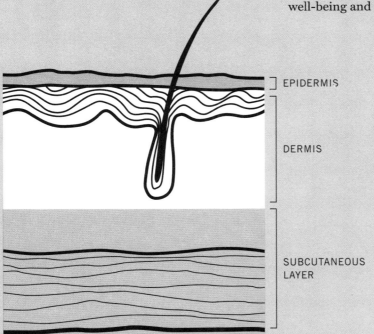

EPIDERMIS

DERMIS

SUBCUTANEOUS
LAYER

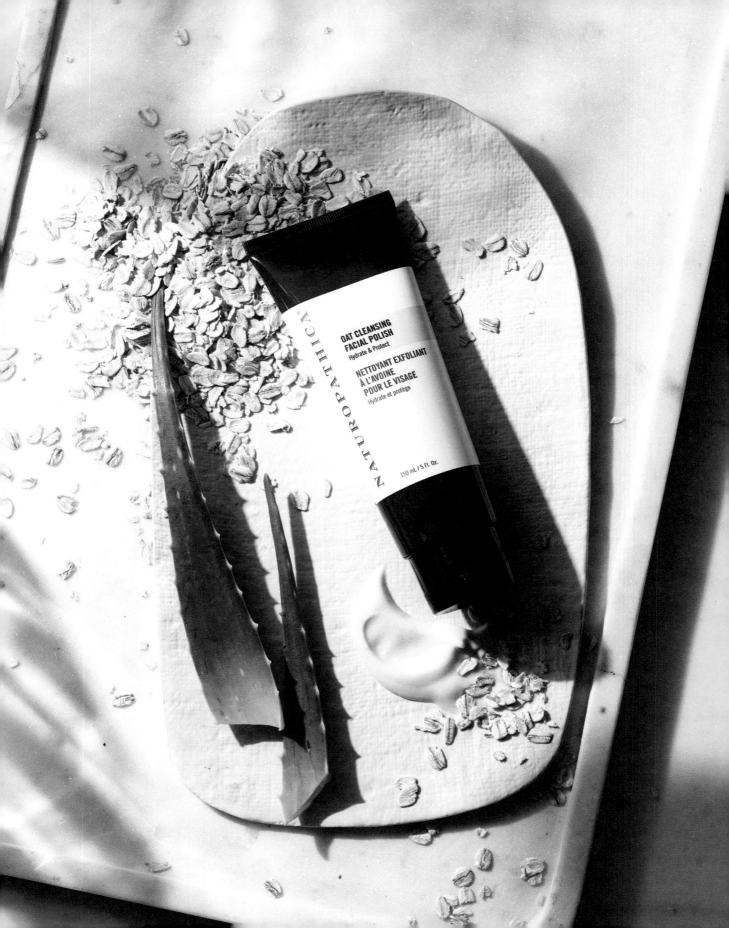

Step 2: Slough

Exfoliation is the second-most important step in skin care. Your skin constantly regenerates itself from the bottom up. Skin cells begin in the dermis as round, plump, compact cells, but as they follow their journey upward, they become irregular and less compact and firm, finally shedding off the surface of the skin. In our twenties, this naturally occurring process takes about 30 days, but when we reach our fifties, it takes double that amount of time, leading to a buildup of dead cells that gives the skin a rough texture. This not only contributes to a dull complexion; the buildup can also block pores and promote breakouts.

Regular exfoliation is one of my favorite beauty rituals, because by removing dead skin cells and product buildup, we can accelerate the making of fresh, healthy new cells to create a dewy complexion. Also, the reality is, there is no point investing in expensive serums or moisturizers if you have a layer of dead skin cells glued to the surface of your skin. Save your money, as the products won't penetrate the skin effectively.

The secrets are to not overdo it and to use the right exfoliant. Below are some of my favorite methods for exfoliation. Note: When using any exfoliant, an SPF must be applied daily.

Mechanical Exfoliation It's likely the skin scrubs you are most familiar with are "mechanical" versions, which you use to physically rub the dead skin cells off, like those inexpensive, coarse apricot scrubs from the drugstore. Avoid those, as the irregular surface particles tear at the skin and actually promote irritation. Look for exfoliating "spheres" or "beads" to gently wick away dead skin cells—but only natural ones, such as jojoba beads, which are biodegradable and will not pollute our waterways. You can also use a soft face brush to exfoliate, paired with a rich cleansing balm to remove product buildup and stimulate microcirculation. Fortified with skin-soothing ingredients, both can be used daily for a glowing complexion.

Enzymatic Exfoliation Fruit enzymes are a step up from mechanical exfoliation, as they penetrate the skin more deeply and act as little Pac-Men, breaking down the protein bonds that hold dead skin cells together. Not only will you get a deeper peel, but the aromatic bouquet from the fruit pulp makes for an intoxicating beauty ritual; do it two or three times a week. Look for pear enzymes to renew the skin, pumpkin to detoxify, or cherry to brighten.

Hydroxy Acids (AHA and BHA) Alpha hydroxy acids (AHAs) are derived from various sources, such as sugarcane to form glycolic acid or milk to produce lactic acid. AHAs have a smaller molecule that penetrates the skin more deeply, dissolving the intracellular glue of the epidermis. Beta hydroxy acid (BHA), also known as salicylic acid, is derived from willow bark and is considered one of the best exfoliants for correcting congested skin. Used sparingly, these exfoliants have the added benefit of stimulating new collagen and elastin.

Several of the leading natural skin care companies do not use AHAs or glycolics in their product lines because they feel that this exfoliation is not a "natural" process internally generated by the body. I have never understood this controversy. There are many physiological processes of the body that are the result of a causative factor. In fact, that is how many natural therapies work—by provoking a low-grade inflammatory response to induce a therapeutic reaction. For example, eucalyptus oil is an effective expectorant because it induces the lungs to expel phlegm.

Glycolics come in many different strengths, ranging from a 5 percent concentration, which you can buy over the counter at the drugstore, to 30 percent, as in preparations used in dermatologists' offices and other contexts. However, what is important to understand is that it is not the strength of the glycolic but the pH level that makes it effective in softening the skin. Generally, the lower the pH level, the stronger the glycolic. Make sure to avoid any glycolic product that uses butylene glycol as a penetration enhancer, because butylene glycol is a known irritant and is the last thing to which you want to expose your freshly cleansed skin.

Step 3: Treat

Now that you have prepared your palette, so to speak, by removing a layer of dead skin cells, it's time to treat the skin with a serum or concentrate. Unlike moisturizers, these powerful formulas do not contain oil and have smaller molecules to penetrate the deepest layers of the skin with a high concentration of antioxidants, vitamins, and minerals. If you are in your thirties or older, this step will make a huge difference towards improving the look of your skin. Skin serums are often formulated with ingredients like vitamin C, salicylic acid, or retinols to address specific problems such as sunspots, oiliness, firmness, or fine lines and wrinkles. Concentrates are supercharged formulas with a higher percentage of actives that are designed to be used for a limited amount of time, and work to address specific skin concerns including breakouts, lack of radiance, signs of aging or dryness.

Although it may seem counterintuitive, there is absolutely nothing wrong with putting high-quality oils on your face (yes, even if you have an oily complexion); they do not cause breakouts.

Step 4: Fortify

All skin is thirsty. More specifically, every skin personality is in need of strengthening the skin barrier to protect it from internal free-radical damage as well as external environmental aggression from things like UV light and pollution. In the brick wall metaphor (see page 19), your skin begins to lose the mortar that holds the bricks in place, leaving gaps and irregular spaces that are ripe for infection or inflammation. Moisturizers infuse the skin with beneficial ingredients to help maintain the structure of the wall.

One way you can fortify and protect your skin is by using a facial oil. When Naturopathica introduced facial oils at our healing arts center and spa in 1995, many of our clients were skeptical about using oil on their skin—until they saw the results. Today it's so exciting to see facial oils become legitimized as part of an effective skin care regimen. Although it may seem counterintuitive, there is absolutely nothing wrong with putting these high-quality oils on your face (yes, even if you have an oily complexion); they do not cause breakouts. Because oils have a small molecular structure, they are more easily absorbed into the skin than creams, thus quickly and thoroughly delivering their healing benefits.

Unfortunately, many commercial facial oils contain base oils that have been extracted using a synthetic solvent such as hexane. Residues from such solvents irritate the skin and can cause breakouts and rashes. Cold-pressed vegetal and nut oils are a healthier alternative. Since these oils are not heated extensively during the extraction process, they contain more healthy vitamins, essential fatty acids, and antioxidants that feed the skin. Perform a Facial Massage (page 81) to help promote circulation, condition the skin barrier, and relax the facial muscles, thereby returning a healthy glow to your skin.

Moisturizing lotions, creams, and balms combine an emulsion of water and oil to help hold more moisture in the skin and to act as a barrier that helps prevent dehydration. Choose a moisturizer according to the amount of oil in your skin (oily complexions will want a more fluid lotion while dry skin types will need a heavier cream or balm). Keep in mind that depending upon the season or climate, your skin will need more or less hydration at different times. Apply moisturizer after a bath or shower while the skin is still damp, or mist your face with a floral water or hydrolat to increase water permeability.

What sets a holistic facial apart from a standard deep-cleansing facial is the stimulation of the body's own natural healing systems, and the treatment of the cause of the imbalance rather than the symptom. Here is what to expect from a holistic facial:

Consultation and Analysis Expect the esthetician to not only ask about your needs and goals for the session but to also inquire about diet, stress level, and skin care regimen to identify the nutritional as well as the lifestyle factors that may be influencing your skin.

Cleansing Stimulation The lymphatic system is part of the body's immune and waste-disposal system and consists of a network of fluid-filled vessels distributed throughout the body under the surface of the skin. During the cleansing phase, the esthetician will use lymphatic brushing or massage techniques to mechanically stimulate the flow of lymph, aiding the lymph nodes to filter out impurities.

Massage Stimulation A good facial massage should not only stimulate circulation and release endorphins but also relax the muscles of the face, neck, and shoulders to reboot the nervous system.

Education Your esthetician will teach you that it takes more than just applying moisturizers to have healthy skin. Radiant skin begins within and is achieved by eating the right foods and embracing the restorative properties of plant medicine, healthy sleep habits, and well-being rituals.

Step 5: Sun Survival

The facts: There is no such thing as a safe tan. Tanning is just as harmful as a burn. Some sunlight is essential for both our physical and emotional well-being, but excessive exposure to the sun causes the skin's collagen to break down, immediately prompting an inflammatory response in the body. Sun exposure also causes wrinkles and dark spots, and can lead to a leathery texture as the skin works to build up a thicker outer layer to protect the body.

Be smart: Make applying sunblock part of your daily regimen, even in winter. And this is important, too: a physical block is always superior to chemical sunscreens. Only a natural full-spectrum sunblock such as titanium dioxide or zinc oxide will block out both UVA and UVB rays, as these compounds act as a physical barrier on the skin which deflects the harmful elements, thereby preventing cellular damage. You may have found that physical sunblocks are harder to rub in than chemical-based sunblocks like octyl methoxycinnamate or Parasol, but be patient. New formulations have made these sunscreens easier to absorb, and the benefits are worth it, as synthetic sunblocks are loaded with skin-irritating ingredients.

As we all know and feel, we have both physical and emotional needs for sunlight. Our bodies absorb sunlight through the skin and convert its properties as part of the process of making vitamin D, which is necessary for the proper absorption of calcium, in addition to other vital functions. Chronic vitamin D deficiency has long been associated with rickets, a softening and weakening of the bones, but more recently and increasingly, scientists are discovering that vitamin D is important in preventing a host of health problems, from muscle and joint aches to skin imbalances such as atopic dermatitis, acne, or rosacea. Sunlight provides the vital energy that supports all life on this planet, just one powerful element of which is the sensual warmth of sunlight that is essential to our emotional balance. Ensure you get adequate exposure to sunlight, but again, be smart. Apply sunblock to your face and enjoy sunbathing the rest of your body when you can for about 20 minutes before 9 a.m., when the sun's rays will not burn. After that, make sure you apply enough sunblock to cover exposed areas—use 1 ounce (enough to fill a shot glass) for the entire body, and reapply every 2 hours.

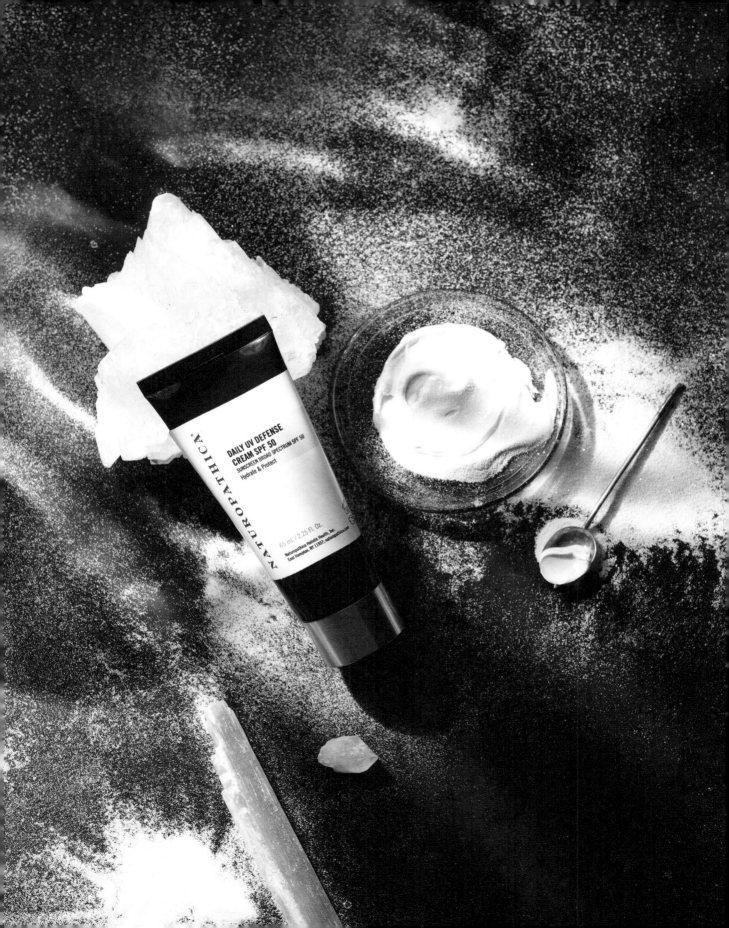

Step 6: Put Your Best Face Forward

While in the past, spas were a place for a day of luxurious rest and relaxation, today top spas focus less on pampering and more on teaching clients about health and well-being with results-oriented treatments. These skin care centers employ top estheticians (and sometimes dermatologists as well) to get your skin looking its best.

Find a good spa in your area and, if you can, have a facial at least four times a year, with the change of the seasons (see the Resources section on page 153 for a list of Naturopathica spa partners specializing in holistic skin care). A good facial goes a long way towards flawless skin. An esthetician can give you a deeper cleansing, exfoliation, and massage than you can give yourself at home. However, if you are on a budget, of course at-home facials are an option as well; study proper techniques and locate the right products—or make your own—with the help of resources like this book.

There are some essentials you need to look for in a good facial. You want high-quality products with botanical ingredients and clean base materials that support the integrity of the skin. A good esthetician will do a comprehensive intake form and also address the main cleansing systems of the body, the lymphatic and circulatory systems.

Step 7: Sleep

They don't call it beauty sleep for nothing. Make sure you get at least 7 to 8 hours of sleep most nights. If sound sleep is a problem for you, explore some of the remedies on page 127.

Step 8: Everything in Moderation—Even Moderation

Cigarette packs in Europe carry the following warning statement: "Smoking kills. Stopping smoking reduces the risk of fatal heart and lung diseases." That gets right to the point. Simply put, smoking is horrible for the skin as well, starting with causing premature aging by depriving the cells of oxygen.

As for other vices, I am the last one to discourage a good glass of wine. But remember that alcohol dehydrates the skin and is loaded with sugar—which, if you remember, is like gasoline for inflammation. If hard liquor is your poison, stick to small amounts of dry, clear spirits like gin, vodka, and tequila, which are very low in fructose. Surprisingly, wine contains very minimal amounts of fructose, but avoid champagne or dessert wines. Beer, unfortunately, contains a lot of sugar, so its low-alcohol content is not a good trade-off, or at least be aware. And always remember to balance alcohol intake with lots of water: follow every glass of alcohol you consume in the course of an evening with two glasses of water. On those nights when you lose a little control, drink a liter of water before your head hits the pillow.

There are some essentials you need to look for in a good facial. You want high-quality products with botanical ingredients and clean base materials that support the integrity of the skin.

Step 9: Work It Out

Second only to diet in maintaining healthy skin, exercise does more for your skin than any skin care cream will. Exercise gives all of your organs a surge of oxygen, and your skin benefits especially, since oxygen increases collagen production as well as hydration and prevents free-radical damage. Working out promotes the cleansing of the blood by stimulating circulation and robust perspiration, which also aids the skin microbiome.

Researchers now believe that even small amounts of exercise, undertaken in short bursts of intense effort followed by a slightly longer recovery time, not only uses more calories but also improves aerobic fitness and burns more fat. This adaptive response is very powerful and, as we will see in the discussions in later chapters about herbal remedies, the phenomenon kicks the body's cellular-maintenance functions into high gear.

Step 10: The Stress-Less Step

You find yourself racing toward home while inhaling a slice of pizza behind the wheel, or arguing with your mother-in-law on the phone at work while analyzing a spreadsheet before a critical meeting. Figured out yet how to master that stress-free lifestyle? You must be joking.

But stress is no joke: Prolonged stress promotes the release of the hormone cortisol in the body, which is a major contributor to numerous health problems including reduced immunity, insomnia, fatigue, and cognitive impairment. And our skin, because it interacts with the circulatory, nervous, and immune systems, as well as reacting to emotional swings, often manifests its own set of skin-related problems such as acne, eczema, hives, psoriasis, and rosacea when we are stressed.

While stress may be an inevitable part of our busy lives, how we adapt to stress is not. It is important to use all of the self-care resources, routines, education, and disciplines we can find to address stress, whichever and however we can make them fit our schedules. Always try to be aware of your stress levels and strive to keep them within healthy limits to avoid imbalances. Chapter 5 of this book (page 124) explores ways to regroup and rebalance in order to mitigate the effects of stress.

Chapter 2

Customized Beauty Rituals
for Your Skin Personality

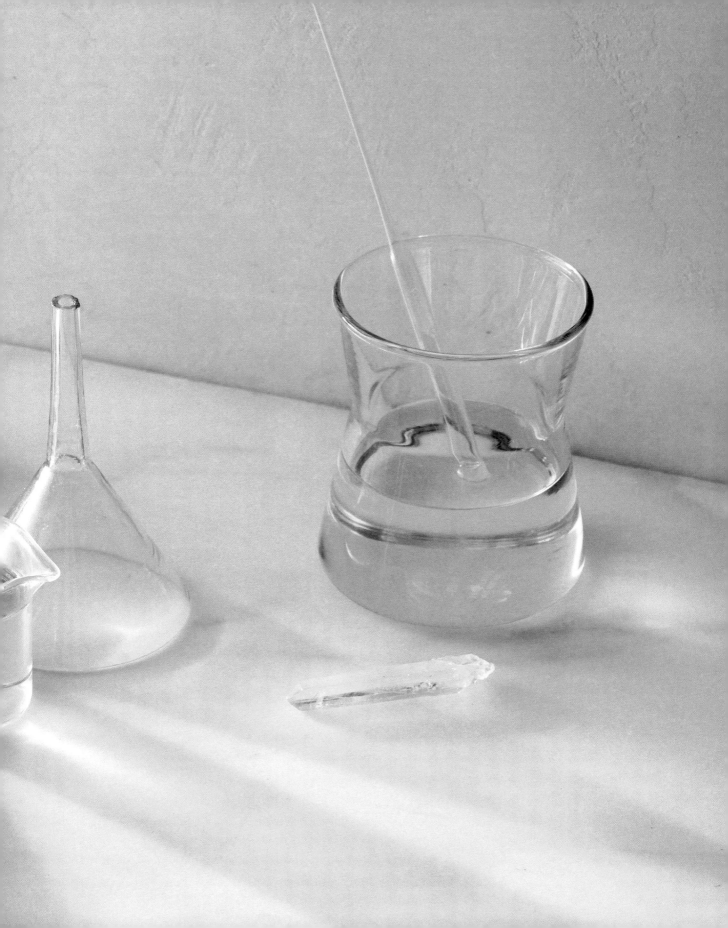

Holistic skin care stipulates that every individual has their own unique skin profile and, accordingly, a beauty ritual that can be prescribed to achieve optimal health and performance. Starting with general descriptions and brief checklists, the following section will help you identify which of four main skin personality categories your individual profile falls into, and then provides detailed guidelines for regimens, remedies, diet, supplements, and suggestions to help you care for the needs of your particular skin from the inside out.

Skin Personalities

In the late 1960s, a trend toward "scientific" skin care led to a definition of the skin types that many of us still think of today as the big three: normal, dry, and oily. This more or less academic—or anecdotal—classification system went on to dominate the skin care industry and essentially changed how women looked at their skin. Even today, your skin type is often determined by how much or how little oil your skin produces, using that outdated classification system, which in rough terms breaks down as:

Normal Medium-sized pores, smooth skin tone
Oily Enlarged pores, shiny skin, prone to blemishes
Dry Small pores, skin feels tight, some flaking

The reasoning behind this classification system is that by knowing your skin type, you can better understand how to help to minimize irritation and help to correct problems.

Skin-typing, while a useful topical diagnostic tool, is overly simplistic and does not tell the whole story of how or why a person's skin has become imbalanced. Oily or dry skin is not just a genetically given complexion, but is the result of a systemic imbalance within the body and thus begs the question, what are the causative factors that have given rise to this condition? The cause may have multiple origins, such as hormones or nutritional deficiencies, and until the cause has been addressed, the condition cannot be effectively treated.

A holistic approach to well-being and beauty always looks at symptoms from an in-depth perspective, since symptoms are simply messages that the body is sending us. I prefer to call my classifications "skin personalities" instead of "skin types" because I think this brings a perspective that more accurately reflects how our bodies work—in particular, our skin as a living, communicating organ. By my thinking, these skin personalities can be broken down into four main groups, as follows.

A holistic approach to well-being and beauty always looks at symptoms from an in-depth perspective, since symptoms are simply messages that the body is sending us.

A   ADAPTIVE

I have always disliked the skin-type label "normal," because it implies that everyone who does not fit that description is somehow inadequate (are they "abnormal"?). Adaptive skin is resilient or balanced skin that requires minimal attention; concerns are resolved quickly. Over 75 percent of men and women fall into this category.

HR   HORMONE REACTIVE

This skin personality is somewhat mercurial, more actively driven by the ebb and flow of hormones. At the time of a woman's menstrual cycle, the hormones that impact the skin are mainly sex hormones called androgens, which stimulate the sebum glands to enlarge, make more oil, and clog the pores. During menopause, estrogen, along with its anti-inflammatory properties, drops dramatically, giving rise to sensitive skin, rosacea, and allergies. Hormone reactive skin tends to have enlarged pores, excessive oiliness, and blemishes, and is prone to sensitivity.

SR   STRESS REACTIVE

Stress creates havoc in our bodies. It causes our adrenal glands to work overtime, producing excessive amounts of cortisol, which raises our "fight or flight" response and eventually results in adrenal fatigue. Taxing our endocrine system can lead to decreased immunity, circulatory problems such as high blood pressure, insulin resistance, sleep disturbances, and skin imbalances. Stress reactive skin is more likely to exhibit the impact of the external forces that bear down on it: changes in temperature, sunlight, humidity, and allergens all have a direct effect on the clarity of the skin. Blemishes, rosacea, dermatitis, eczema, and psoriasis are all exasperated by stress. Stress reactive skin has an average pore size and moderate oil production (mainly in the T-zone) but is highly sensitive to factors such as lack of sleep, poor diet, a high-pressured lifestyle, and changes to the environment.

M   MATURE

Despite the huge number of antiaging treatments on the market, the truth is that time does the same thing to everyone: it ages the skin. Certainly, there are factors that can hasten this process, for example, overexposure to sunlight, smoking, and chronic inflammation. Mature skin is thin, lacks moisture and may show facial lines, wrinkles, and sun damage.

**DO ANY OF THE
FOLLOWING TRAITS
APPLY TO YOUR SKIN?**

☐ Average pore size

☐ Oiliness and/or dryness
in the T-zone

☐ Uneven tone or sun damage

☐ Occasional congestion,
breakouts, milia, or cystic
bumps

☐ Occasional dull complexion
or uneven texture

☐ Occasional symptoms
of fatigue, indigestion,
colds/flus

SKIN CARE REGIMEN

`Cleanser` Adjust your cleansing regimen as needed, using a sulfate-free, gel-based cleanser when your skin is in an oily phase and a cream cleanser during a dry phase. Wash once or, if necessary, twice a day. Look for botanicals such as aloe, oats, lavender, rose, or German chamomile to help strengthen the skin barrier and calm inflammation. Try the Clarifying Cleansing Oil on page 73.

`Exfoliant` Use a fruit enzyme peel like the **Naturopathica Pear Fig Polishing Enzyme Peel** or an alpha hydroxy acid peel 2 to 3 times a week to revitalize a dull complexion, or try the Cleansing Facial Gommage on page 74.

`Toner` Use a facial mist with herbs such as aloe or lavender to adjust the pH of your skin and soothe it after cleansing and exfoliating. Try the Green Tea Toner recipe on page 75 and a compress with lavender (see page 130).

`Serum, followed by a Facial Oil` Treat your skin after exfoliation with an active serum made with ingredients like plant stem cells or marine extracts such as *Fucus serratus,* a supercharged antioxidant with a high vitamin content. When used topically, these ingredients help treat and prevent oxidative damage. Follow with a lightweight facial oil made with a base of vegetal oils such as jojoba or borage seed, which are rich in gamma-linolenic acid, an essential fatty acid needed in collagen production (see page 59). Try the Neroli Toning Facial Oil on page 78.

`Moisturizer` Look for a light- to medium-weight moisturizer containing antioxidants such as vitamins A, C, and E as well as soothing herbs that support the skin barrier such as beech tree, calendula, and gotu kola. Always apply a sunblock, ideally with minerals such as zinc, a physical barrier as well as a natural antiseptic, and skin-soothing herbs such as lavender before going outdoors.

SKIN FITNESS

While nutritional deficiencies are often less a factor for adaptive skin, your skin will still thank you for focusing on the Beauty Foods listed on page 101 and doing the 14-Day Detox Plan (page 107) in spring and fall to cleanse and renew the body.

HERBAL REMEDY CHEST

Herbal Infusions Begin your day with a Rosemary-Lemon Beauty Tonic (page 141) to alkalinize your body upon waking. Drink 2 to 3 cups of Skin Tea (page 145) daily, a mixture made with green tea (an antioxidant) fortified with calendula, lemon balm, and lavender to soothe the skin and relax over-stressed nerves.

Herbal Tinctures A healthy gut is essential for radiant skin. Add 2 dropperfuls of an herbal tincture (a liquid herbal extract; see page 147) made with liver-cleansing herbs such as milk thistle, yellow dock, and/or dandelion root to a glass of water or tea and take before meals in the morning and evening.

Topical Remedies Apply tea tree oil directly onto your skin with a cotton swab to help clear up occasional breakouts.

SUPPLEMENT SUPPORT

Take a multivitamin that includes A, C, and E to slow down oxidative damage (especially if your diet is not balanced). Supplement with 1000 IUs daily of vitamin D3 to promote remineralization.

BEAUTY & BALANCE

Incorporate more relaxing rituals into your days. Purchase an aromatherapy diffuser (see Resources, page 153) and try diffusing essential oils, at home or work, to promote relaxation. Begin or end your day with a 20-minute yoga and meditation ritual to help ground emotions. Try the Grounding Breath exercise on page 133.

SKIN CARE Rx

Boost your skin with a reviving face mask once a week to replenish your complexion; try the Avocado-Honey Mask on page 83.

Try a "facial sauna" (see the Clarifying Facial Sauna on page 74) to help remove impurities.

Give yourself a facial massage with your choice of serum twice a month (see page 81).

Begin your day with a lavender compress (see page 130) to boost circulation.

Deflate puffy eyes in the morning by soaking black tea bags (rich in caffeine) in water and placing over your eyes for about 5 minutes.

Get a professional holistic cleansing facial (see page 24) every 3 to 4 months, if you can.

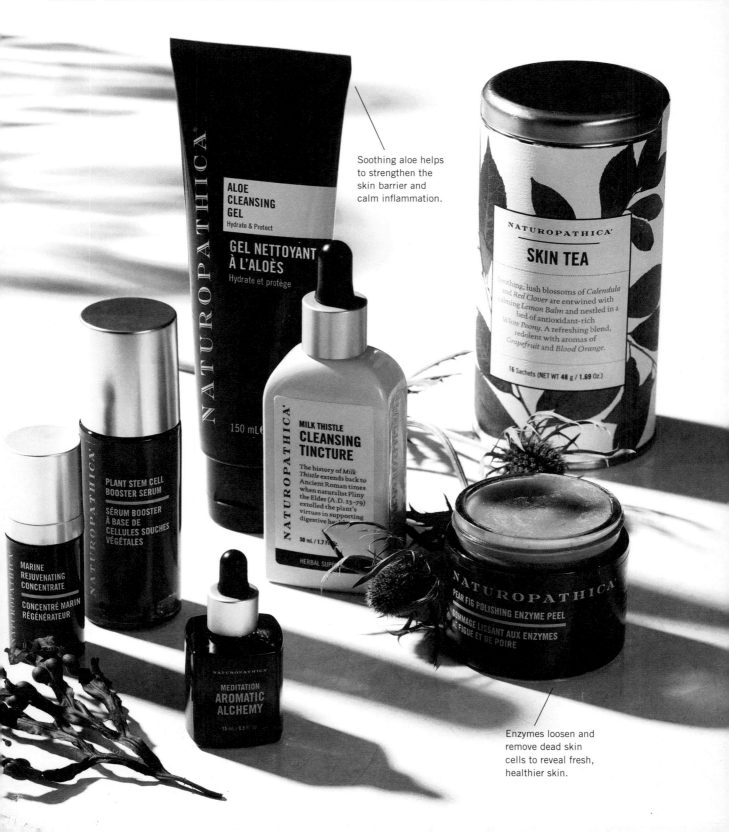

Soothing aloe helps to strengthen the skin barrier and calm inflammation.

Enzymes loosen and remove dead skin cells to reveal fresh, healthier skin.

Promote radiant skin from the inside out by sipping tea fortified with antioxidants and soothing herbs.

SKIN CARE REGIMEN

Cleanser Use a sulfate-free, gel-based cleanser once or twice (but no more) a day to combat oiliness. Look for antiseptic herbs such as tea tree, cypress, and juniper to keep skin clear, as well as skin-soothing aloe vera, since breakouts are a sign of inflammation.

Exfoliant Keep pores clear with an enzyme peel such as pumpkin, or try the Cleansing Facial Gommage on page 74. For blemished skin, exfoliate daily with a glycolic containing salicylic acid (derived from willow bark) to unclog pores or excess oil and to accelerate cell turnover.

Toner Use a facial mist with antiseptic herbs like lavender, or try the Clarifying Parsley Toner recipe on page 76.

Serum or Facial Oil Look for a serum with a high percentage of salicylic acid (to clean out congested pores) as well as hyaluronic acid (HA). Found naturally in the skin, HA guards against inflammation, calms sensitivity, and holds in moisture—critical factors since most hormone reactive skin is dehydrated. Use a lightweight facial oil with a base of slightly astringent vegetal oil (see page 59) such as marula, and combine with antiseptic essential oils such as rosemary, tea tree, and lemon. Try the Blemish Facial Oil on page 79.

Moisturizer Use a lightweight or oil-reducing moisturizer with antioxidants such as vitamins A, C, and E. Make sure any product you're considering does not contain acne-exacerbating oils such as lanolin, mineral oil, or other petroleum-based ingredients; instead, look for skin-soothing aloe or hyaluronic acid to calm irritation along with antiseptic herbs such as rosemary and lemon to tone the skin. Once menopause arrives, look for moisturizers with vitamin A (retinol) or peptides to stimulate collagen production. Always apply a sunblock (preferably physical; see page 24) to skin before going outdoors.

SKIN FITNESS

Sugar is particularly bad for hormone reactive skin, as it is inflammatory and increases blood glucose, which in turn increases insulin, thus triggering androgen activity and sebum production.

Avoid dairy, as it also is inflammatory. For menopausal skin, try to include soy-based foods such as tofu or soy milk in your diet; these contain phytoestrogens (i.e., plant estrogens such as isoflavones), which can help to regulate the effects of estrogen and modulate dryness and sensitivity.

Pack your diet with the Beauty Foods listed on page 101, and include a focus on cruciferous vegetables (broccoli, cauliflower, cabbage, Brussels sprouts, and kale, to name a few), which can help detoxify the body and balance hormone levels. Cruciferous vegetables are unique sources of sulfur-rich compounds called glucosinates that support liver detoxification by triggering antioxidant and anti-inflammatory responses in the body.

Incorporate more fermented foods, such as sauerkraut or kimchi (see the recipes on pages 119 and 120) in your diet.

HERBAL REMEDY CHEST

Herbal Infusions Drink a shrub, a traditional herbal beverage of fruit syrup blended with apple cider vinegar, to boost good bacteria; to make your own, try the Black Cherry and Cardamom Shrub on page 142. If you prefer a warm drink, see the Golden Turmeric Latte on page 145. Research suggests that not only does turmeric have many anti-inflammatory benefits and supports good gut health, it also plays a role in preventing several chronic diseases including Alzheimer's disease, arthritis, and cancer.

Herbal Tinctures Add 2 dropperfuls of an herbal tincture (a liquid herbal extract; see page 147) made with skin-clarifying herbs such as burdock root, Oregon grape root, or dandelion to a glass of water or tea and take before morning and evening meals.

Topical Remedies Apply aloe vera to overreactive skin to calm inflammation. For menopausal skin, apply evening primrose oil, a good source of gamma-linolenic acid, directly to the skin to soothe dryness and sensitivity. Apply tea tree essential oil or moss extract directly onto your skin with a cotton swab to help clear up breakouts.

SUPPLEMENT SUPPORT

Take a multivitamin daily. In addition, take 30 to 60 milligrams of zinc. Research indicates that zinc reduces inflammation and also inhibits androgens that promote acne.

BEAUTY & BALANCE

Incorporate some stress-reducing activities such as aerobic exercise or yoga into your daily routine, or soak in a relaxing herbal bath dosed with clary sage essential oil, an herb possessing estrogen-like qualities and used to ease premenstrual symptoms (See Aromatherapy Blending on pages 66). Or, try a relaxing Prana Ear Massage (page 129).

SKIN CARE R_X

Do not over-wash your skin; this can cause oil glands to overcompensate.

Do not "pop" pimples. But since you are going to be tempted to do this anyway, here's how: Using clean hands wrapped in cotton or tissues, gently squeeze blackheads. Sweep away any debris and dab with tea tree oil or hydrogen peroxide.

Make a Purifying Green Tea Mask (page 83) and apply for 10 minutes to draw out impurities and soothe sensitive skin.

Mist your face with antiseptic facial mist or toner throughout the day to keep your skin bacteria free.

Get help: Schedule regular monthly facials to help control breakouts and target problem areas with extra-strength peels and treatment serums.

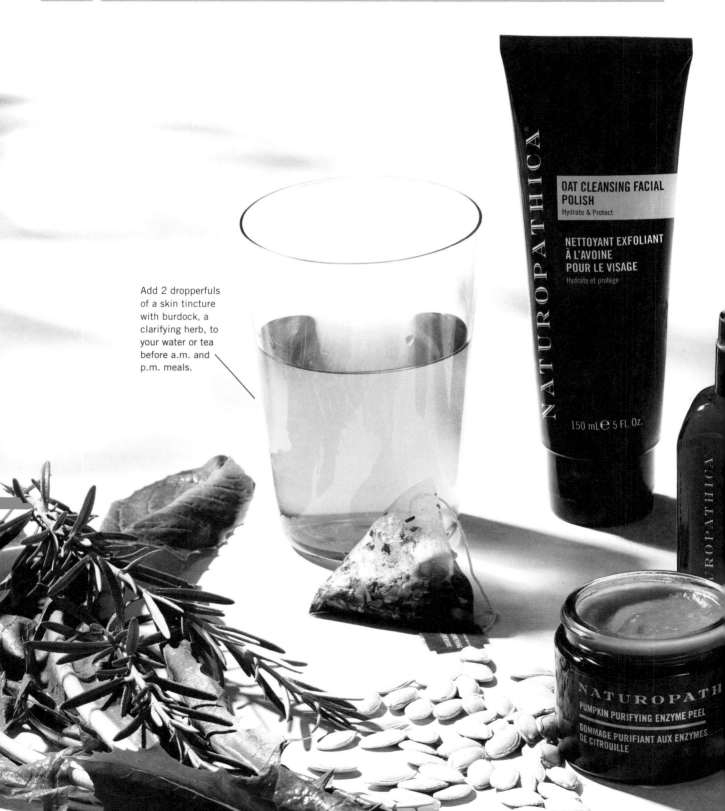

Add 2 dropperfuls of a skin tincture with burdock, a clarifying herb, to your water or tea before a.m. and p.m. meals.

NATUROPATHICA®

OAT CLEANSING FACIAL POLISH
Hydrate & Protect

NETTOYANT EXFOLIANT À L'AVOINE POUR LE VISAGE
Hydrate et protège

150 mL℮ 5 Fl. Oz.

NATUROPATHICA

NATUROPATHICA
PUMPKIN PURIFYING ENZYME PEEL
GOMMAGE PURIFIANT AUX ENZYMES DE CITROUILLE

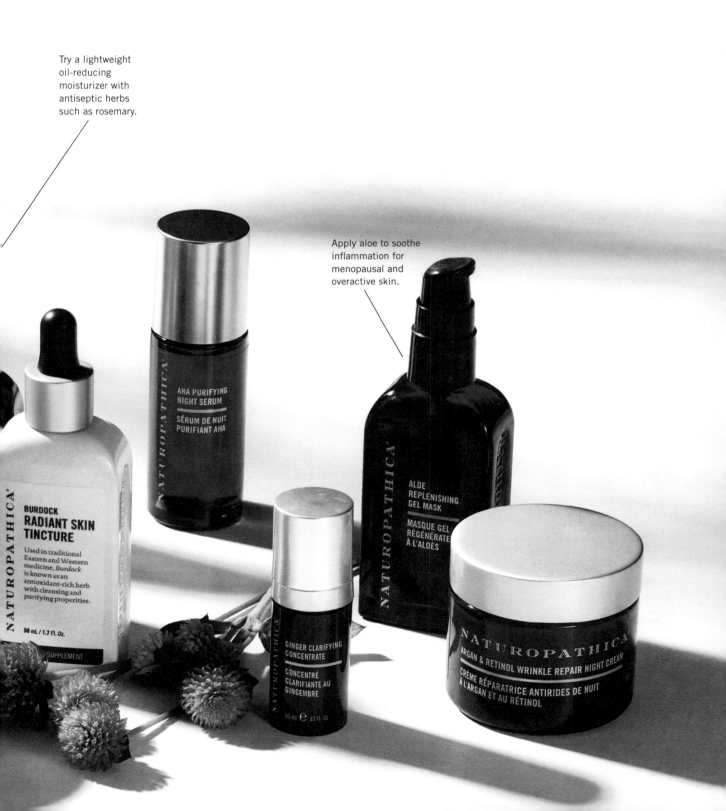

Try a lightweight oil-reducing moisturizer with antiseptic herbs such as rosemary.

Apply aloe to soothe inflammation for menopausal and overactive skin.

NATUROPATHICA

BURDOCK
RADIANT SKIN
TINCTURE

Used in traditional
Eastern and Western
medicine, *Burdock*
is known as an
antioxidant-rich herb
with cleansing and
purifying properties.

50 mL / 1.7 FL Oz.

SUPPLEMENT

NATUROPATHICA

AHA PURIFYING
NIGHT SERUM

SÉRUM DE NUIT
PURIFIANT AHA

NATUROPATHICA

GINGER CLARIFYING
CONCENTRATE

CONCENTRÉ
CLARIFIANTE AU
GINGEMBRE

10 mL ℮ .33 FL. Oz.

NATUROPATHICA

ALOE
REPLENISHING
GEL MASK

MASQUE GEL
RÉGÉNÉRATEUR
A L'ALOÈS

NATUROPATHICA

ARGAN & RETINOL WRINKLE REPAIR NIGHT CREAM

CRÈME RÉPARATRICE ANTIRIDES DE NUIT
À L'ARGAN ET AU RÉTINOL

**DO ANY OF THE
FOLLOWING TRAITS
APPLY TO YOUR SKIN?**

☐ Moderate oiliness, mostly
in T-zone area

☐ Breakouts during stressful
periods or changes in
temperature or humidity

☐ Small blemishes, usually
localized around mouth
and chin area

☐ Episodic patches of red,
rashy skin or flaky, dry skin,
especially on face, hands,
feet, or elbows

☐ Family history of psoriasis,
eczema, hives, or other
skin imbalances

☐ Occasional or frequent headaches, cold sores, allergies,
asthma, or indigestion

SKIN CARE REGIMEN

Cleanser Use a sulfate-free cleanser with anti-inflammatory herbs such as aloe and chamomile once a day, or try a rich cleansing balm with humectants like mango butter and honey to draw moisture to the skin. Look for fermented ingredients like *Lactobacillus* ferment or yogurt to help good bacteria to flourish.

Exfoliant Do not exfoliate during reactive phases when rashes or itching are present. During dormant phases, exfoliate the skin with fruit enzymes like papaya or pear, or try the Cleansing Facial Gommage on page 74.

Toner Calm down irritated skin with a rose facial mist, or try the Plant Milk recipe on page 76.

Serum or Facial Oil Replenish your skin with a serum using plant stem cells—potent antioxidants to promote wound-healing—and hyaluronic acid to boost moisture. Use a medium-weight facial oil with a base of vegetal oils such as argan, avocado, and evening primrose, rich in nutri-ents and beneficial for skin barrier repair. Look for soothing and cell-regenerating essential oils like carrot seed, rose, or lavender to add to the base oil. Try the Carrot Seed Protective Facial Oil on page 79.

Moisturizer Use a rich moisturizer containing calming ingredients such as aloe vera, calendula, or borage seed oil as well as antioxidants like vitamins A, C, and E. Make the Healing Calendula Balm on page 138 to soothe dry, irritated skin. Always apply sunblock, preferably with a physical-blocking mineral such as zinc and a soothing herb like lavender, before going outdoors.

SKIN FITNESS

Watch out for foods that may cause an inflammatory response in the body, such as the sugary and high-glycemic foods you may be more attracted to during stressful periods (see pages 94–95). Avoid red meat, dairy, and spicy foods, which are acid-forming and may help create heat in the skin, thus aggravating skin imbalances. Eat raw oats, such as muesli, with coconut milk for breakfast instead of oatmeal, as cooked oats are acid-forming. Ramp up on skin-loving omega-3 fatty acids, found in wild salmon, nuts, and seeds. Eat more of the "good fats" (monounsaturated) such as avocados and olives, which are also high in antioxidants. Do the 14-Day Detox Plan (on page 107) twice a year to cleanse the system from stress-related eating or anytime the skin becomes red, scaly, and itchy for a prolonged phase (see Food Sensitivities, page 95).

HERBAL REMEDY CHEST

Herbal Infusions Begin your day with a Rosemary-Lemon Beauty Tonic (page 141) to alkalinize your body upon waking. Drink 2 to 3 cups of Stress Tea (page 147) daily, a mixture made with adaptogen herbs, including schisandra berry and holy basil, to build resistance to stress by balancing cortisol.

Herbal Tinctures Research suggests that Oregon grape root may be helpful for aggravated skin conditions such as psoriasis or eczema.[1] For daily prevention, supplement with adaptogen herbs such as Siberian ginseng or schisandra to boost immunity and energy reserves as well as support overtaxed adrenal glands. In acute conditions, look for sedative herbs such as skullcap, passionflower, or oats, traditionally used as tonics for the nerves, to help calm overstimulated nerves frayed from itching. All of these herbs can be ingested as an herbal tincture (see page 147) that can be added to hot water, juice, or tea.

Topical Remedies Oats help to balance skin pH and also help soothe and repair the skin barrier. Make the Plant Milk on page 76 and spritz throughout the day. Follow with the Healing Calendula Balm on page 138.

SUPPLEMENT SUPPORT

Take a multivitamin daily. In addition, take 500 mg black currant oil in the morning and evening to calm down dry, red, aggravated skin. Black currant oil contains gamma-linolenic acid (GLA), an omega-6 fatty acid that promotes healthy growth of skin. You should begin to notice positive changes in 6 to 8 weeks.

BEAUTY & BALANCE

Because stress and cortisol play a big role in inflammation, try to incorporate some of the stress-balancing techniques outlined in Chapter 4, such as the Relax Herbal Bath on page 132. Create your own calming aromatherapy blend with essential oils such as lavender, neroli, geranium, or rose using the blending guidelines on page 67. Apply to pulse points to help rebalance the mind and body throughout the day.

SKIN CARE Rx

Avoid hot showers and baths when your skin is aggravated. Try to bathe once a day in cool water, getting in and out and as quickly as possible so as not to strip the body of precious oil. Apply a thick moisturizing cream immediately after patting yourself dry.

Look for skin-soothing herbs such as aloe vera, calendula, gotu kola, or burdock in creams or balms to calm irritated skin.

Sleep is the best antidote for stress reactive skin types. Drink a relaxing herbal tea such as chamomile or lavender before bed and keep an herbal tincture with passionflower, valerian, and/or kava by your bedside in case you wake up in the middle of the night. Review the sleep tips on page 127.

If your skin becomes irritated frequently, buy a pH test kit at your drugstore to determine the acidity of your body. Acid-forming foods create skin disturbances such as rashes, hives, or intense itching (see page 95).

Fortify your skin with extra omega-3 fatty acids to calm down skin during especially stressful times: take 500 milligrams of evening primrose oil or black currant oil twice daily.

Add an herb-infused honey with adaptogens Siberian ginseng and schisandra to build resistance to stress.

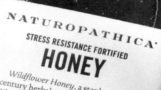

NATUROPATHICA®

STRESS RESISTANCE FORTIFIED

HONEY

Wildflower Honey, a staple of the 19th century herbal medicine chest, is infused with *Siberian Ginseng, Ginger Root* and *Ginkgo*, along with spicy *Cinnamon, Clove* and *Cardamom* to restore strength and vitality.

95 mL / 3.3 Fl. Oz.

HERBAL SUPPLEMENT

NATUROPATHICA

CHIL
AROM
ALCH

15 mL /

NATUROPATHICA

CARROT SEED
SOOTHING
FACIAL OIL

HUILE APAISANTE
POUR LE VISAGE
À LA GRAINE DE
CAROTTE

NA
CALENDU

CRÈME HYD
À LA CALENDU

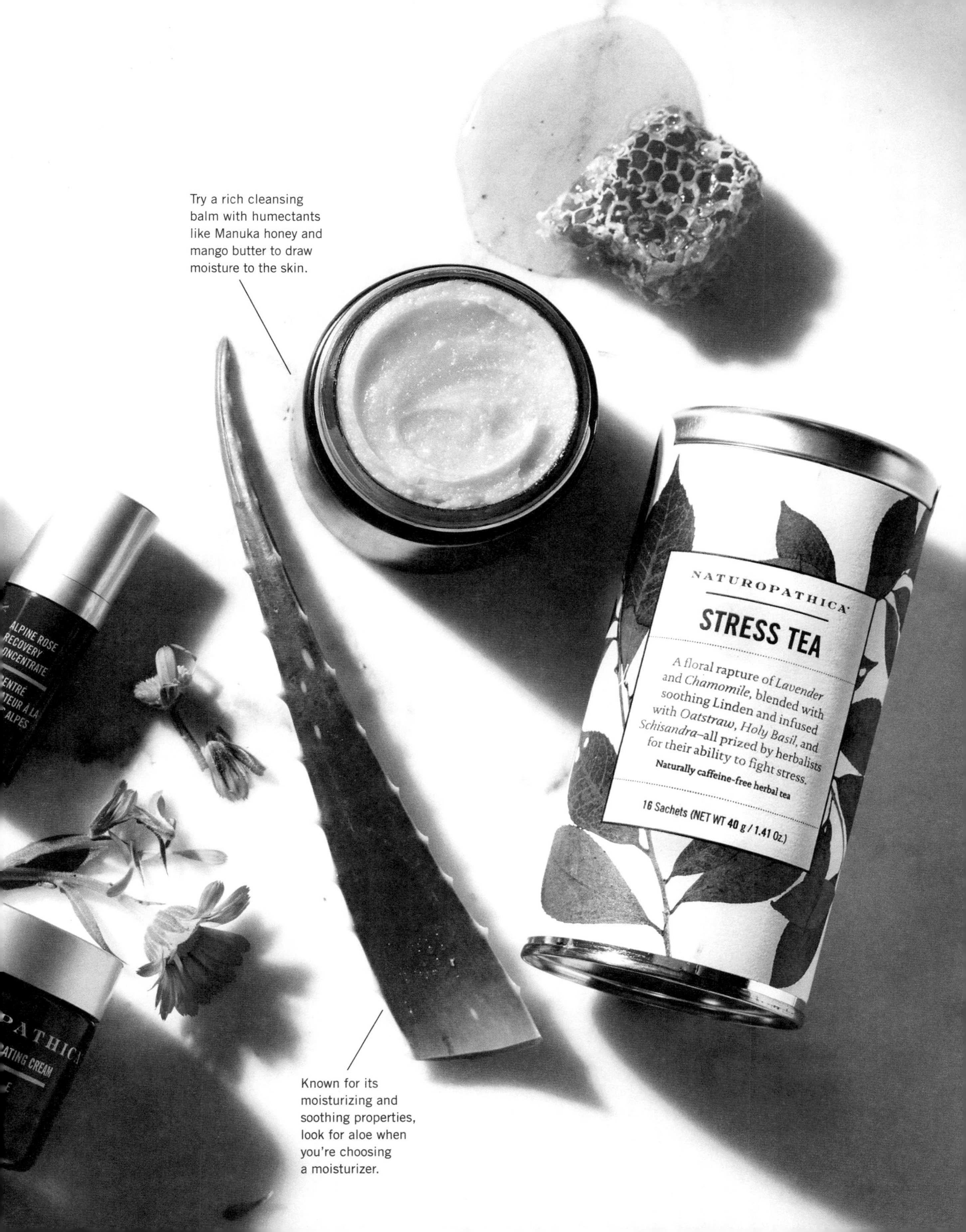

Try a rich cleansing balm with humectants like Manuka honey and mango butter to draw moisture to the skin.

ALPINE ROSE
RECOVERY
CONCENTRATE

CENTRE
ATEUR À LA
ES ALPES

NATUROPATHICA®

STRESS TEA

A floral rapture of *Lavender* and *Chamomile*, blended with soothing Linden and infused with *Oatstraw, Holy Basil,* and *Schisandra*—all prized by herbalists for their ability to fight stress.

Naturally caffeine-free herbal tea

16 Sachets (NET WT 40 g / 1.41 Oz.)

PATHICA
ATING CREAM

Known for its moisturizing and soothing properties, look for aloe when you're choosing a moisturizer.

**DO ANY OF THE
FOLLOWING TRAITS
APPLY TO YOUR SKIN?**

- ☐ Less/minimal oil production
- ☐ Wrinkles, dark spots, and/or discoloration
- ☐ Thinner and drier epidermis (see page 19)
- ☐ Loss of firmness
- ☐ Broken capillaries, especially on nose and cheeks
- ☐ Occasional or frequent bruising, bloating, weight-gain, or insomnia

SKIN CARE REGIMEN

Cleanser Use a soothing, sulfate-free cream cleanser once a day with hydrating herbs like German chamomile or sweet lupine, or try a rich cleansing balm with humectants like glycerin and honey to draw moisture to the skin.

Exfoliant Do a regular exfoliation program several times a week using an enzyme peel with antioxidant ingredients such as sweet cherry or an alpha-hydroxy acid (unless your skin is sensitive, look for a 10 percent glycolic acid).

Toner Use a rose geranium facial mist, or try the Plant Milk recipe on page 76.

Serum or Facial Oil Replenish the skin with an antioxidant serum containing plant stem cells or vitamin A to stimulate cell turnover. Also look for vitamin C to lighten skin hyperpigmentation. Use a heavier-weight facial oil with a base of rich vegetal oils such as rose hip, evening primrose, or baobab fortified with a high percentage of essential fatty acids to support collagen synthesis. Supplement facial oil with anti-inflammatory and skin-regenerating essential oils such as everlasting, lavender, or geranium. Try the Geranium Regenerating Facial Oil recipe on page 80.

Moisturizer Use a rich moisturizer containing skin-hydrating ingredients such as hyaluronic acid and oat beta glucan (derived from oatmeal) as well as peptides to stimulate the cell fibroblasts to produce collagen. Apply a thin layer of a hydrating mask to your face and leave on overnight to give your skin a moisture surge. Rinse off with tepid water in the morning. Always apply sunblock, preferably a physical block (see page 24) with minerals such as zinc, a natural antiseptic, and skin-soothing herbs such as lavender before going outdoors.

SKIN FITNESS

A proper diet is key for healthy, mature skin. Cruciferous vegetables are especially beneficial for mature skin, since they are potent detoxifiers for the liver. Focus on foods rich in omega-3 fatty acids, which help skin cells maintain water and resist irritation. Omega-3s can be found in oily fish such as salmon, sardines, or mackerel, as well as grass-fed animals and free-range eggs. Consider making a Beauty Bone Broth (page 122), rich in collagen that will help keep the skin plump, or a Sea Mineral Broth (page 123), which remineralizes the body with magnesium, calcium, and iron. Do the 14-Day Detox Plan (page 107) in the spring and fall to cleanse and renew the body.

HERBAL REMEDY CHEST

Herbal Infusions Begin your day with a Rosemary-Lemon Beauty Tonic (page 141) to alkalinize your body upon waking. Follow with a daily cup of Moringa Matcha Latte (page 144), packed with antioxidants to fight free-radical damage.

Herbal Remedies Add 2 dropperfuls of an herbal tincture (a liquid herbal extract; see page 147) made with calming herbs for frayed nerves such as holy basil and passionflower to a glass of water or tea and take before meals in the morning and evening.

Topical Remedies Facial oils penetrate the skin deeper than most creams, and for older skin this is a must. Select a facial oil or serum fortified with essential fatty acids to plump up your skin and do a Facial Massage (page 81) once a week.

SUPPLEMENT SUPPORT

Take a multivitamin daily. Take 500 milligrams of borage seed or evening primrose oil, rich in gamma-linolenic acid, to help counteract oxidative stress to the skin.

BEAUTY & BALANCE

Healthy, radiant skin manifests when stress is low, so make sure you take time out to nurture yourself—you've earned it. Find new ways to stimulate your mind and support your creative energies, such as traveling, reading, or starting a new hobby. Spend a weekend alone at a spa or yoga retreat. Experiment and try a new activity.

SKIN CARE Rx

Older skin needs more nourishment: Add a rich cleansing balm to your cleansing ritual 2 to 3 times a week to infuse the skin barrier with more nutrients.

Buy a humidifier for your bedroom to let your skin recharge with 8 hours of sufficient moisture every night. Be sure to clean the filter regularly and add a calming essential oil to the water to help you relax.

Mix 2 drops of a facial oil or serum with your moisturizer for an extra boost to feed your skin.

Put a thin layer of a hydrating mask on your face and leave on overnight. Rinse off with tepid water in the morning to give your skin a moisture surge.

Mature skin has sluggish cell turnover. Keep a regular schedule of monthly holistic facials to give your skin the extra care it needs with professional-strength AHA peels.

Use a soothing sulfate-free cream cleanser with hydrating sweet lupine once a day.

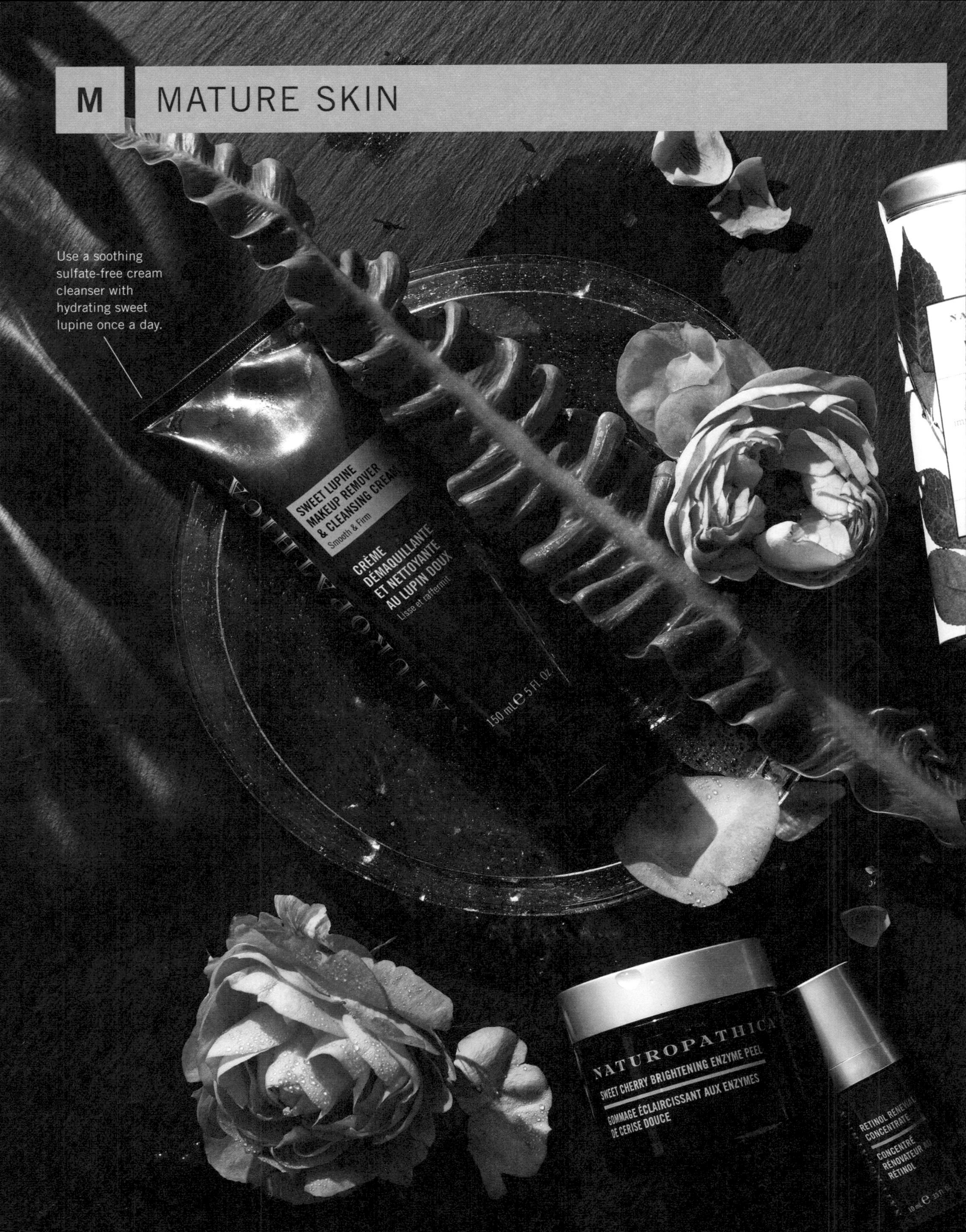

SWEET LUPINE
MAKEUP REMOVER
& CLEANSING CREAM
Smooth & Firm

CRÈME
DÉMAQUILLANTE
ET NETTOYANTE
AU LUPIN DOUX
Lisse et raffermit

150 mL ⊖ 5 FL OZ

NATUROPATHICA

SWEET CHERRY BRIGHTENING ENZYME PEEL

GOMMAGE ÉCLAIRCISSANT AUX ENZYMES
DE CERISE DOUCE

RETINOL RENEWAL
CONCENTRATE

CONCENTRÉ
RÉNOVATEUR
RÉTINOL

To help ease frayed
nerves, add 2 dropper-
fuls of an herbal
tincture with calming
oats and passionflower
to water or tea before
a.m. and p.m. meals.

NATUROPATHICA

OATS
**STRESS RELIEF
TINCTURE**

According to
King's American
Dispensary, the
19th-century book
of herbal medicine,
Oats are considered
a restorative nerve
tonic for exhaustion.

50 mL / 1.7 Fl. Oz.

HERBAL SUPPLEMENT

NATUROPATHICA

RE-BOOT
AROMATIC
ALCHEMY

15 mL / 0.5 Fl. Oz.

NATUROPATHICA

DAILY UV DEFENSE
CREAM SPF 50
SUNSCREEN BROAD SPECTRUM SPF-50
Hydrate & Protect

65 mL / 2.25 Fl. Oz.

Naturopathica Holistic Health, Inc.
East Hampton, NY 11937 naturopathica.com

Apply a chemical-free,
physical sunblock with
zinc oxide and fortified
with antioxidants like
green tea extract
before going outdoors.

Chapter 3

Pure Ingredients,
Pure Results

Skin Care Recipes

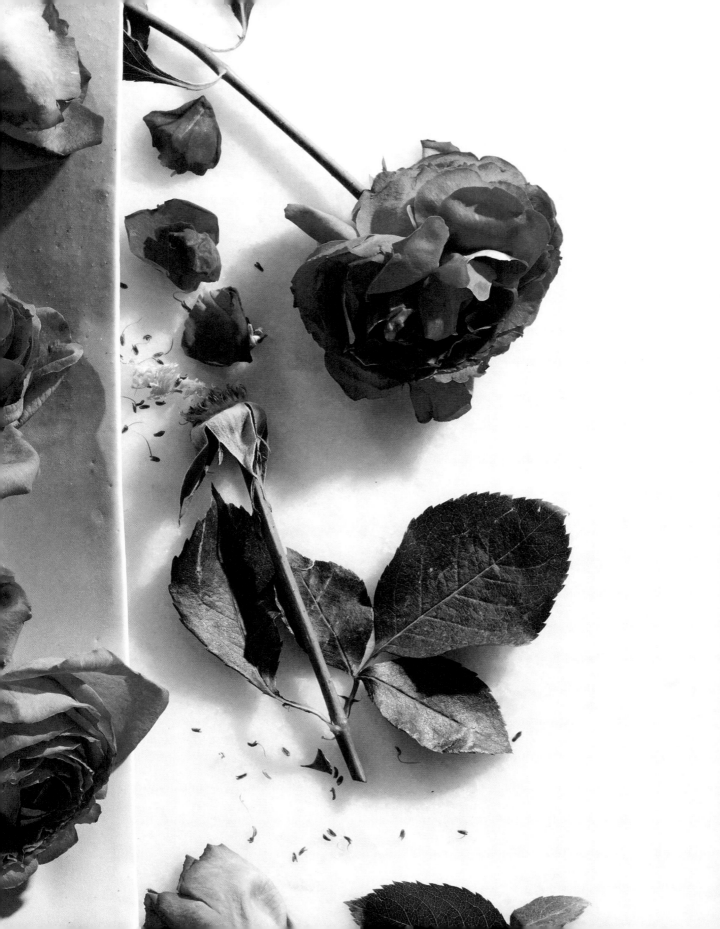

One way to ensure you are buying products that are safe for you and the environment is to look for certified cosmetic products. Naturopathica products are certified by ECOCERT, which upon its introduction in 2003 was the first certification body to develop standards for natural and organic cosmetics. Now there are dozens of others—NaTrue, Cosmebio, and the USDA, to name a few.

Unfortunately, certifications can be confusing, so another thing to look for is if a brand uses INCI labeling. The International Nomenclature of Ingredients is an internationally recognized labeling system that companies adopt voluntarily to identify ingredients. Learning about these certification bodies and knowing your ingredients empowers you with a greater understanding of your skin and helps you limit your exposure to potentially toxic or irritating products.

It isn't easy trying to limit the number of chemicals you put into your body. You try to eat healthy, choosing organic foods and drinking filtered water. But what about all the other chemicals your skin is exposed to every day? Even throughout a seemingly harmless morning routine, our bodies can be exposed to countless chemicals.

Many products that you might typically pick up in the beauty section of a grocery or drugstore can wreak havoc on your skin. Most commercial soaps have a pH of 8 or higher, which creates an alkaline environment that destroys the good bacterial flora of the upper epidermis, making the skin more vulnerable.

Many shampoos and conditioners contain DEA *(diethanolamine)*, MEA *(monoethanolamine)*, or TEA *(triethanolamine)*, most commonly seen on a label as cocamide DEA, which may affect hormone function and can form cancer-causing agents known as nitrosamines.

Facial cleansers often contain sodium lauryl sulfate (or *sodium laureth sulfate)*, a widely used foaming agent and surfactant that is very irritating to the skin and eyes. Most toners are alcohol-based, making them drying to the skin. Many facial moisturizers use a sunscreen with oxybenzone, which can cause skin allergies and may affect hormone function.

All of the examples above demonstrate just how often we unknowingly interact with toxic chemicals every day, and this bad chemistry could be part of the rise in cancer and other diseases.

Savage Beauty

According to Ecovia Intelligence, the global natural and organic skin care market is a $12.6 billion industry and is projected to grow to $22 billion by 2024. North America comprises a $4.7 billion market share.[1] Once restricted to the domain of health-food stores and natural-foods supermarkets, natural personal-care products are no longer niche products and have been mainstreamed, presiding over the aisles at large beauty chains, and even drugstores and mass merchandisers.

When I wrote the first edition of this book ten years ago, I felt the need to include a chapter about the abundance of chemicals in skin care products and raise awareness about their potential for toxicity. "Greenwashing," a modern form of spin whereby organizations use deceptive marketing to create the perception that their products or policies are environmentally friendly, was common in the skin care arena through the practice of adding botanical extracts to cosmetics loaded with synthetic base materials and then pronouncing the product "natural." Slowly, things are beginning to change. In 2004, the Environmental Working Group launched Skin Deep, the first cosmetics database to help consumers find information about the ingredients they are putting on their skin and understand their potential hazards. Today the tides have turned as consumers, particularly millennials, want to see toxic materials replaced, and hold traceability and ethical sourcing of ingredients as an important standard.

INGREDIENTS TO AVOID

NAME	DESCRIPTION
DEA (*diethanolamine*) **MEA** (*monoethanolamine*) **TEA** (*triethanolamine*)	Often appearing on labels as cocamide DEA, these chemicals, derived from coconut oil, are commonly used in cleansers, shampoos, and body washes as an emulsifier and foaming agent. Research suggests these chemicals may cause liver and kidney cancer and disrupt hormone function.
FD&C Color Pigments	Often made from coal tar, these artificial colorings can cause skin sensitivity and may be carcinogenic.
Fragrance	The chemicals used to create artificial fragrances can be very sensitizing to the skin. Many of the synthetic compounds in fragrance are toxic and can cause headaches, dizziness, or nausea.
Hydroquinone	A skin-bleaching chemical. In animal studies, hydroquinone has caused tumor development. It is banned in Japan and the EU.
Imidazolidinyl Urea and DMDM Hydantoin	These preservatives are known to cause contact dermatitis according to the American Academy of Dermatology. They also release formaldehyde, a chemical that can cause skin irritations as well as health problems such as migraines, allergies, and asthma.
Parabens	This widely used class of preservatives was originally developed in the 1930s to stabilize creams. The greatest concern regarding parabens' effects focuses on the possible disruption of hormone function and increased risk of breast cancer. Parabens also increase skin sensitivity.
Petrochemicals	This category includes any petroleum-derived compound, usually identifiable on labels by the prefixes or suffixes such as propyl-, methyl-, eth-, or -ene. Petrochemicals deplete the Earth's resources, are common irritants for many individuals, and do not offer any nutritive benefit to the skin. Two petrochemical ingredients commonly found in skin care products are: **Isopropyl Alcohol** A solvent found in emollients and cleansing agents. **Mineral Oil** This familiar oil is sensitizing to the skin due to residues and contaminants.
Phthalates	This group of chemicals is mainly used in products to increase the softness and flexibility of plastics. The greatest concern focuses on dibutyl phthalate, often found in nail polish, and diethyl phthalate, a common ingredient in skin care lotions, as they may affect hormone function.
Polyethylene Glycol (*PEG*)	Used to break down oil or help thicken products, this ethoxylated wetting compound for detergents, foaming agents, emulsifiers, and solvents is sometimes contaminated with 1,4-Dioxane, a potential carcinogen that can penetrate the skin.
Sunscreen Chemicals	Common sunscreen ingredients PABA, avobenzone, homosalate, methoxycinnamate, and oxybenzone are used for their ability to absorb UV light. However, there is some concern that they may act as endocrine disruptors and also damage cells by allowing UV light to penetrate the skin.

Feeling Sensitive?

While I am happy to see more transparency in cosmetic formulations, I think the next step is to broaden our focus from safety to sensitivity. When we first opened our Healing Arts Center & Spa, Naturopathica East Hampton, about 25 percent of our clients characterized themselves as having sensitive skin. According to a recent 2014 Mintel study, 71 percent of facial skin care users say they are interested in ultra-gentle products.[2]

This is a drastic increase in skin sensitivity, certainly partially due to the increase in environmental pollution that assaults our skin every day. But the rise in sensitive skin is primarily caused by allergenic, irritating ingredients that age the skin prematurely. These ingredients are primarily found in the base materials of many conventional skin care products—the surfactants, emulsifiers, and preservative systems that make up these formulas. And since inflammation is the primary cause of premature aging of the skin, it's important to know which are the main culprits that flame the fires of irritation. Use this list to find and weed out skin irritants that may be lurking inside your medicine cabinet.

- Preservatives linked to health issues and skin irritation (parabens, phenoxyethanol, DMDM hydantoin, diazolidinyl urea, imidazolidinyl urea, BHA and BHT)
- Petroleum or petroleum-derived ingredients (mineral oil, paraffin wax, carbomer, benzene, toluene)
- Animal ingredients (lanolin, musk, collagen, squalene)
- Synthetic fragrances (phthalates, DBP, DMP, DEP)
- Synthetic colors and dyes
- Silicones
- Synthetic polymers (nylon, polyacrylamide, elastomers, poloxamer, styrene, vinyl)
- Synthetic fragrances (phthalates: DBP, DMP, DEP)
- Ingredients hazardous to the environment (non-biodegradable, toxic, harmful: EDTA, silicones, triclosan)
- Hydroquinone
- SLS, SLES, ALES, cocamidopropyl betaine, octoxynols
- 1,4-dioxane, ethoxylated compounds (PEGs, PPG, ceteareth, polysorbate 60, -80)
- Nitrosamines (MEA, TEA, DEA)
- Glycols and diglycols (propylene glycol, ethylene glycol, butylene glycol)
- Quarternary ammonium compounds (polyquaternium)
- Synthetic sunscreens (PABA, oxybenzone, benzophenones)
- Aluminum zirconium

Pure Ingredients

Nature possesses complex and powerful ingredients whose benefits cannot be replicated in a laboratory. Here is an overview of some of those prized natural substances that can truly benefit the skin and help ease some of the causes of inflammation, with no dangerous side effects. These are the building blocks for the skin care recipes throughout this book.

ESSENTIAL OILS

Essential oils, used in aromatherapy, are derived from flowers, leaves, seeds, roots, and resins of aromatic plants to promote health and well-being. Essential oils are highly concentrated substances, often referred to as "the life force of the plant," containing chemical compounds with many antiseptic, antifungal, analgesic, anti-inflammatory, and antiviral properties.

Holistic skin care uses clinical-grade essential oils, genuine natural essential oils that are not compromised by extraction with harsh solvents or adulterated by processing in the laboratory. Over 95 percent of the essential oils produced worldwide today are made for the perfume, food, and taste industries. These synthetic oils have no therapeutic value to the skin and promote skin irritation.

Essential-oil molecules enter our bodies in two main ways: by inhalation or through the skin. (A third route, ingestion, is also practiced in much of Europe, but is not advised unless under the supervision of a qualified herbalist.) Smelling calming scents like lavender or clary sage affects both the limbic system of the brain, the seat of emotions and memory, and also the skin, since stress has a big influence on the health of your epidermis. Because of their unique, small molecular structure and the fact that they are lipid (fat) soluble, essential oils can also penetrate the skin, entering the bloodstream via the capillary network and circulating throughout the body, where they have a systemic effect.

PSYCHOAROMATHERAPY

It's easy to understand why our sense of smell can go far beyond its basic functions to influence the mind and affect behavioral changes in the body. Close your eyes and imagine biting into a ripe, juicy, freshly cut lemon. Do you notice your mouth filling with saliva as your mind envisions the smell and taste of the bitter lemon? The right scents provide a wide range of both uplifting and relaxing responses in the body and can be used as a powerful tool to rebalance the body.

ESSENTIAL OILS

NAME & ORIGIN	PROPERTIES & USES	COMMENTS
Atlas Cedar *Cedrus atlantica*	This rich and warm oil is known for its antiseptic properties, is ideal for blemished skin, and contains stress-relieving properties.	
Balsam Fir *Abies balsamea*	The balsamic and woody aroma of this oil works as an antidepressant, delivering uplifting qualities and working as a decongestant to stimulate circulation.	
Bay Laurel *Laurus nobilis*	This oil stimulates and has a cleansing effect on the lymphatic system.	
Bergamot *Citrus aurantium bergamia*	Typically grown on the southern coast of Italy, this oil's bright, citrus aroma helps ease stress, anxiety, and nervous tension.	Use caution when using bergamot topically as it can increase skin sensitivity and create hyperpigmentation.
Blue Eucalyptus *Eucalyptus globulus*	This oil features a cool and clarifying aroma. Prized for its antiseptic qualities, it can help ease colds, congestion, and muscle stiffness.	
Cardamom *Elettaria cardamomum*	This oil's warm, spicy aroma is grounding and calming, and helps to minimize nausea and constipation.	
Carrot Seed *Daucus carota*	This oil is rich in beta-carotene (vitamin A) and also contains over 50 percent sesquiterpene alcohol, making it useful for skin-cell regeneration and soothing dry, irritated skin.	
Chamomile, German *Matricaria recutita*	A potent anti-inflammatory oil due to high bisabolol content, this oil is excellent for burns or skin inflammations.	The bright blue color is a hallmark of this oil, as is its ripe, honey-apple scent.
Chamomile, Roman *Anthemis nobilis*	A fresh, sweet, apple-like aroma soothes nervous tension, acting as an antidote for stress and anxiety.	
Clary Sage *Salvia sclarea*	This oil's spicy, nutty aroma induces a state of euphoria, ideal for reducing stress and as an antispasmodic for PMS.	
Cypress *Cupressus sempervirens*	Used since ancient times, this smoky and woody oil has grounding benefits and helps to improve concentration.	
Everlasting *Helichrysium talcum*	A high percentage of sesquiterpenes makes this a strong anti-inflammatory oil, excellent for dry, irritated skin or broken capillaries.	A must for every herbal remedy kit, this oil rapidly heals the skin.

NAME & ORIGIN	PROPERTIES & USES	COMMENTS
Frankincense *Boswellia carteri*	The antiseptic and astringent properties of this oil make it useful for toning and clarifying the skin. It's also prized for its skin-cell regenerating properties.	A luxurious and calming scent profile adds to its therapeutic qualities.
Geranium *Pelargonium graveolen*	This oil possesses a combination of terpene alcohols and esters to give it both antiseptic and balancing properties. It also produces a strong relaxing effect on the central nervous system.	This oil is often adulterated, so be sure to purchase from a reputable supplier.
Jasmine *Jasminum sambac*	The sweet and sensuous scent of this oil acts as a heady aphrodisiac and helps reduce nervous tension.	
Juniper *Juniperus communis*	This stimulating oil has antiseptic qualities, making it useful in skin care.	Juniper is an evergreen shrub, the branches of which possess a smoky aroma and were burned by Native Americans to purify the air. The detoxifying and astringent properties of the oil derived from juniper make it great for lymphatic cleansing.
Lavender *Lavandula vera or Lavandula angustifolia*	Lavender comes in many forms and is excellent for toning the skin and promoting relaxation.	Varieties grown in alpine regions of France and Croatia have a high linalool content, making them very antiseptic and especially useful on oily or acne-prone skin or burns. Lowland varieties like those found in the Grasse region of France contain a high ester content, yielding powerfully relaxing oils useful for stress-related conditions.
Lemon *Leptospermum petersonii*	The sparkling and zesty aroma of this oil contributes to its stimulating qualities, which help brighten moods and rejuvenate the mind.	
Lemon Tea Tree *Leptospermum petersonii*	Traditionally used for its antiseptic properties, this uplifting and citrusy oil has cleansing and purifying benefits.	
Neroli *Citrus aurantium*	High linalool, linalyl acetate, and geraniol content give this oil its balancing and soothing properties. It's especially useful in regulating sebum production.	This oil is produced from the small white flowers of the bitter orange tree.
Patchouli *Pogostemon cablin*	The primary use is aromatherapy because of patchouli oil's grounding, earthy scent.	
Peppermint *Mentha piperita*	This oil's sweet aroma has detoxifying properties, providing lymphatic stimulation and acting as an antidepressant to refresh fatigued minds.	

ESSENTIAL OILS

NAME & ORIGIN	PROPERTIES & USES	COMMENTS
Pink Grapefruit *Citrus paradisi*	This oil's sweet aroma has detoxifying properties, providing lymphatic stimulation and acting as an antidepressant to refresh fatigued minds.	
Red Mandarin *Citrus reticulata*	The bright, uplifting scent released by this oil contains stimulating and tonic qualities that relieve stress, anxiety, and nervous tension.	
Rose *Rose Otto damascena*	Citronellal and geraniol give this oil its soothing and balancing properties. Excellent for calming down irritated skin, as well as for relaxing the central nervous system.	An expensive oil to distill due to the large number of rose petals needed to yield a significant amount of the oil.
Rose Geranium *Pelargonium graveolens*	This floral-scented oil has mild antiseptic properties, and is also used to help with mood-balancing.	
Rosemary *Rosmarinus officinalis*	Useful in skin care for its antioxidant and cell-regenerating properties.	Genuine rosemary is usually cultivated in France or Spain and has a high camphor content, making it a great relaxing oil to use in massage.
Sandalwood *Santalum album*	Used since ancient times in ritual practices, this rich and sweet oil has a balsamic, woody scent.	
Sweet Basil *Ocimum basilicum*	The camphorous and spicy aroma of this oil has stimulating and antispasmodic qualities, and helps to promote mental clarity.	
Sweet Lavandin *Lavandula hybrida*	This crisp and bright oil has a calming effect due to its antiseptic properties.	
Tea Tree *Melaleuca alternifolia*	Well-known for its antiseptic and antiviral properties due to a high terpene alcohol content, this oil is beneficial for oily and blemish-prone skin.	Tea tree oil is also useful for the treatment of cold sores, herpes, and nail funguses.
Thyme *Thymus vulgaris*	The *vulgaris* varietal of thyme yields oil that has strong antiseptic qualities but is gentle enough to use on the skin to treat impurities.	

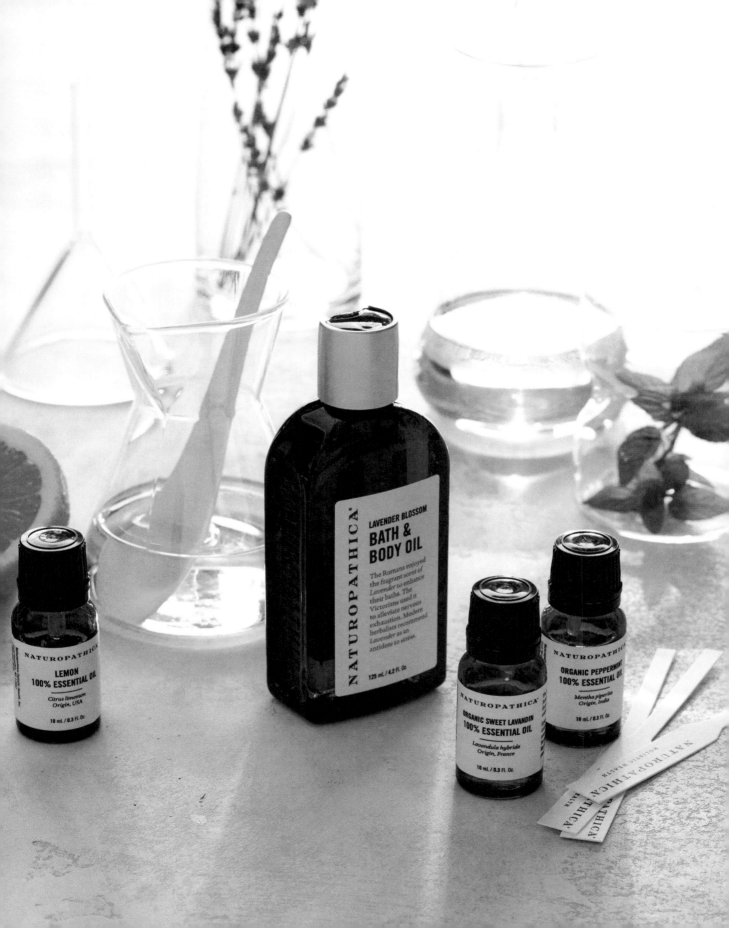

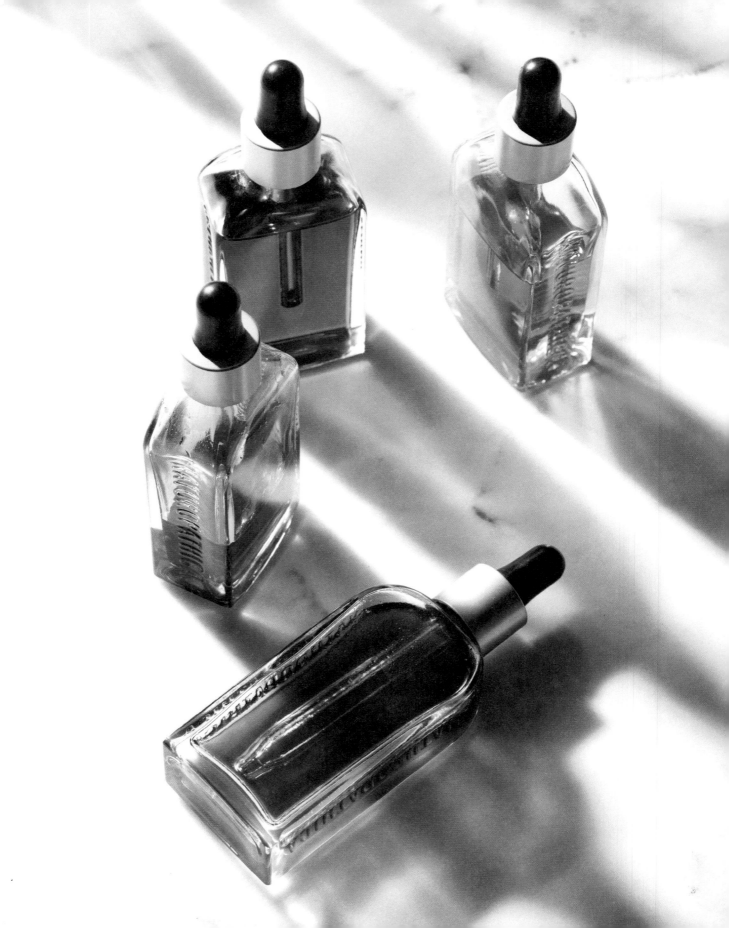

VEGETAL OILS

Carrier oils are an important element in therapeutic aromatherapy and skin care. Due to their high concentration, essential oils need to be diluted in a "carrier," or base, oil before they are applied to the skin. But a carrier oil does much more than just act as a vehicle to deliver essential oils to the skin—it can make all the difference between a low- and high- quality skin care product.

A mineral oil, petrolatum, or paraffin wax can do the job satisfactorily—and very inexpensively. However, these by-products of petrochemical industry processing are inert carriers that are very often irritating and provide no nutritional benefit to the skin. In contrast, vegetal oils, made from nuts and seeds such as argan, sunflower, and borage, offer a wide spectrum of nutritional benefits to the skin, starting with helping to strengthen the membranes that support the cell structure. Remember, the stronger the skin-cell membrane is, the more likely it will be able to protect against inflammation.

The nut or seed of the plant contains the future potential of the plant, its life force. In order for a plant to grow, it must have energy. Seeds and nuts contain this energy in the form of vegetable fats and oils, which they store to make fuel. Vegetal oils also contain many organic compounds that enhance skin function and heal the body, such as essential fatty acids (EFAs)—in particular, omega-3 (alpha-linolenic acid), omega-6 (linoleic acid), and omega-9 (oleic acid). EFAs are polyunsaturated fatty acids necessary for many body functions, especially healthy skin, but our bodies cannot manufacture them. As we will see in Chapter 3, a diet rich in anti-inflammatory EFAs is important for healthy skin, and topical application is key for preserving the fluid lipid coating on the skin's surface. This film holds moisture while protecting against harmful bacteria and pollution, and is in need of reinforcement as the lipid barrier decreases with age.

To make your own high-quality skin care products using vegetal oils, you'll need to make sure the oils have been processed correctly. The best vegetal oils are cold-pressed—that is, produced by heating them gently at low temperatures so that excessive heat does not kill off valuable elements of the oil. In addition, chemical extraction, the use of a petroleum mixture or a solvent like hexane, is not used to render quality oils, as by its very nature, the process changes the effectiveness of the oil. It is common practice in the cosmetic industry to extract vegetal oils with highly pressurized temperatures and with solvents, as this is a shorter process and yields a less expensive oil, so source your ingredients carefully.

TOPICAL APPLICATION OF ESSENTIAL FATTY ACIDS (EFAS)

Topical application of oil is an effective means of delivering EFAs to the skin and strengthening the skin barrier. Because a significant portion of ingested EFAs may be oxidized by the liver (up to 60 percent of alpha-linolenic acid and 20 percent of gamma-linolenic acid) before reaching the skin, topical application may be a more efficient route of delivery.

Omega-9: Oleic Acid Oils high in oleic acid are full-bodied, heavier, and will seal in moisture effectively, making them a good choice for people with dry skin—although some, such as hazelnut and macadamia, can feel lightweight. Oleic acid is known to reduce inflammation.

Omega-6: Linoleic Acid Oils rich in linoleic acid are lighter and thinner in consistency and do not clog pores. Linoleic acid is the most abundant EFA in the epidermis and helps to strengthen the skin barrier. It is useful for inflammatory conditions such as acne, eczema, and psoriasis.

Omega-3: Alpha-Linolenic Acid Derived from fish oils as well as nuts, omega-3 fatty acids help to maintain skin elasticity and also possess anti-inflammatory benefits.

VEGETAL OILS

NAME	PROFILE HIGHLIGHTS	PROPERTIES & USES	COMMENTS
Apricot Kernel	*Linoleic acid: 25–30%* *Oleic acid: 70%*	Rich fatty acid content helps devitalized skin. Light texture good for face serums, especially for oily skin.	Can be used undiluted.
Argan	*Linoleic acid: 30–36%* *Oleic acid: 43–49%*	Used in the beauty rituals of Berber women of Morocco for centuries, this oil is brimming with EFAs and vitamins A and E. Its light texture is great for all skin types.	Use as an addition to a base oil, at 10% of the whole.
Avocado	*Linoleic acid: 6–18%* *Oleic acid: 65%*	The flesh of this fruit yields emollient, full-bodied oil, good for dry, devitalized skin.	Use as an addition to a base oil, at 10% of the whole.
Baobab	*Linoleic acid: 25–34%* *Oleic acid: 30–40%*	Extracted from the fruit of the renowned "Tree of Life" in Africa, this oil is a a power-house, with high levels of vitamin C (six times more than oranges) as well as vitamins A and B for skin elasticity.	
Black Currant Seed	*Linoleic acid: 48%* *a-Linolenic acid: 17%*	The high linoleic (omega-6) and gamma-linolenic content (omega-3) strengthen the skin barrier.	
Borage Seed	*Linoleic acid: 30–40%* *Oleic acid: 18%*	The seeds in this oil, rich in linoleic acid (omega-6), are ideal for aggravated skin conditions such as eczema, as well as for stretch marks and prematurely aged skin.	Use as an addition to a base oil, at 10% of the whole.
Calendula *(infused in sunflower oil)*	*Linoleic acid: 69%* *Oleic acid: 18%*	Traditionally a wound-healing herb, this oil is good for inflamed skin.	Use as an addition to a base oil, at 10% of the whole.
Coconut	*Linoleic acid: 1–3%* *Oleic acid: 5–10%*	Rich, emollient thickener for creams and bases. Look for unrefined, unprocessed oil.	Use as an addition to a base oil, at 10% of the whole.

NAME	PROFILE HIGHLIGHTS	PROPERTIES & USES	COMMENTS
Evening Primrose	*Linolenic acid: 65–75%* *Oleic acid: 8%*	A rich omega-6 profile makes it indispensable in skin care, especially for mature or dry, irritated skin.	Use as an addition to a base oil, at 10% of the whole.
Hazelnut	*Linolenic acid: 17%* *Oleic acid: 74%*	This unique, finely textured oil is highly penetrative despite being high in oleic acid. Good for face serums, especially for oily skin.	Can be used undiluted.
Jojoba	*Oleic acid: 11%*	The flesh of this fruit yields emollient, full-bodied oil, good for dry, devitalized skin.	Can be used undiluted, but is usually used at 30% of the whole.
Macadamia	*Linolenic acid: 3%* *Oleic acid: 60%*	This light, penetrating oil is ideal for face serums. Palmitoleic acid helps delay skin aging with its essential fatty acid content.	Can be used undiluted.
Marula	*Linolenic acid: 7%* *Oleic acid: 75%*	This light-textured oil from the South African tree is rich in vitamins C and E, making it excellent for free-radical protection.	
Rose Hip Seed	*Linoleic acid: 47%* *a-Linolenic acid: 28%* *Oleic acid: 14%*	This is a superb cell-regenerative oil due to its high EFA content. Excellent for scar-healing or for prematurely aged skin.	Use as an addition to a base oil, at 20% of the whole.
Sea Buckthorn	*Linoleic acid: 7%* *Oleic acid: 28%*	The bright red color signals that this oil is rich in antioxidant beta-carotene; it has a good amount of vitamin C as well, and helps ease skin irritation and promote healing.	
Sunflower	*Linoleic acid: 62–70%* *Oleic acid: 20%*	This oil is most commonly used as the base for macerated oils. It has a light texture, similar to human sebum.	Use as an addition to a base oil, at 10% of the whole.
Tatamu	*Linoleic acid: 30%* *Oleic acid: 41%*	Strong antiseptic and anti-inflammatory properties make this a good protective oil.	Can be used undiluted. Suitable base oil for body massage.

HERBAL EXTRACTS

Extracts can be made from a variety of plants, herbs, flowers, and sea plants and are usually derived from an alcohol or glycerin base. These extracts are very concentrated and can have a variety of therapeutic properties. Following are some of the best herbal extracts for skin care.

NAME	PROPERTIES & USES	COMMENTS
Aloe Vera	Aloe contains 95% water as well as minerals, amino acids, proteins, and polysaccharides, therefore making it a valuable humectant and healing agent for burns.	Research shows aloe stimulates the Langerhans cells of the skin's immune system, helping to protect against infection and inflammation.
Green Tea	Potent antioxidant protects skin against the harmful effects of UV exposure, including redness, premature aging, and cancer.	Research shows that topical application of green tea, rich in polyphenols, reduces skin inflammation and neutralizes free radicals, as well as protecting the skin from UV radiation.
Honey	A natural humectant, honey also has antioxidant and mildly antiseptic qualities.	
Licorice Root	A natural anti-inflammatory that helps fight the breakdown of hyaluronic acid, a primary hydrating agent in the skin, and also reduces UV sun damage.	Contains glabridin, a potent antioxidant and skin-soothing ingredient, ideal for stress reactive skin.
Nettle	An herbal infusion useful for its anti-inflammatory properties in healing rashes and burns.	
Oat Beta Glucan	A super-moisturizer similar in efficacy to hyaluronic acid, as it forms a thin, invisible film on the skin to help retention of moisture within. It also has excellent anti-inflammatory properties.	
Plant Stem Cells	Derived from areas of new growth in plants such as the buds or roots, plant stem cells are an exciting new plant-cell-culture technology.	Research supports that several plant stem cells, including those from plants such as echinacea, argan, and butterfly bush, protect the skin from inflammation and environmental stress.
Red Wine	The extract is rich in resveratrol, an antioxidant free-radical scavenger that stimulates cellular proliferation and collagen synthesis.	
Sea Algae	This extract contributes its healing properties to excellent moisturizers that leave the skin feeling smoother, and may cause a significant protective thickening of the epidermis.	Has antioxidant and skin-soothing properties.
Shea Butter	A natural fat obtained from the nuts of the shea (karate) tree in Central Africa, shea butter has a softening effect on the skin and counteracts dehydration.	A rich source of antioxidants as well as skin-replenishing (linoleic) fatty acids.
Turmeric	This botanical extract has strong antioxidant and anti-inflammatory properties, inhibiting the promotion of free radicals on the surface of the skin.	Helps prevent the production of melanin and protect against sun damage.

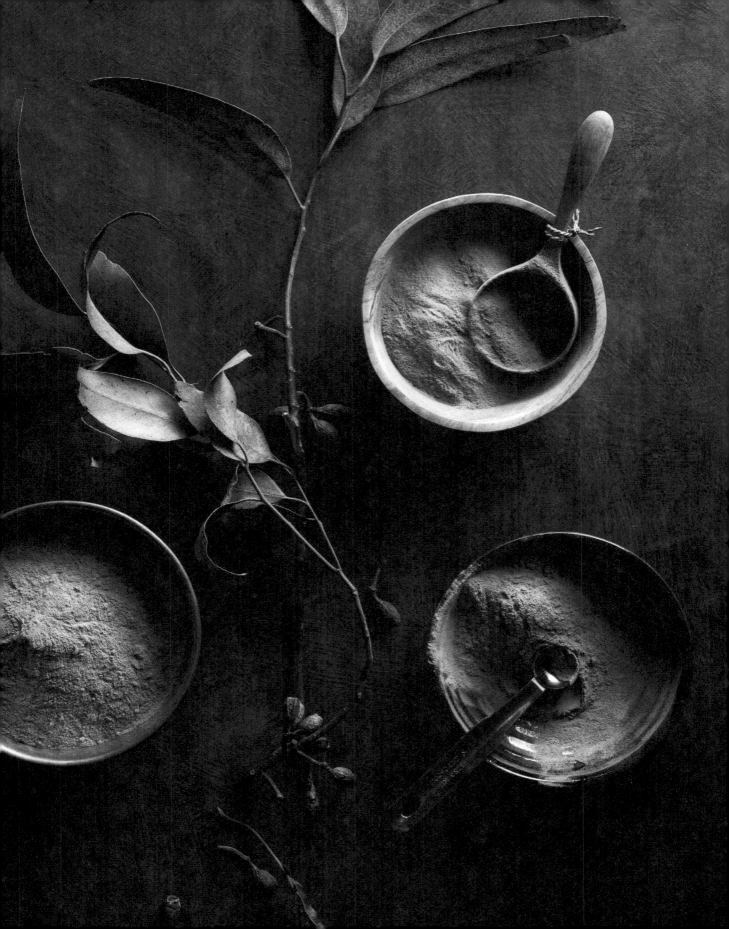

- ☐ Atomizer sprayer
- ☐ Blender or food processor
- ☐ Coffee filters (unbleached)
- ☐ Colored glass bottles, in assorted sizes
- ☐ Double boiler (or saucepan with Pyrex or metal bowl)
- ☐ Food scale
- ☐ French coffee press
- ☐ Glass or ceramic jars with lids, in assorted sizes
- ☐ Grater
- ☐ Hand whisk or immersion blender
- ☐ Measuring cup
- ☐ Mixing bowls (large and small)
- ☐ Mortar and pestle
- ☐ Muslin (cheesecloth)
- ☐ Strainer
- ☐ Tea kettle

Skin Food: Making Your Own Skin Care Preparations

This next section focuses on making your own skin care products. Having summarized the individual components above, now we'll dig deeply into the building blocks and then move on to a comprehensive array of recipes for making your own custom-designed skin care products right in your own kitchen.

Making your own cosmetics at home can be both easy and fun, and has the huge added benefit of allowing you to know exactly what you are using on your skin. You will discover that these recipes do not have to be complicated in order to be effective. All you need is some basic equipment and a handful of supplies easily found at your local hardware, grocery, or health-food store or online (see the Resources section on page 153).

RAW MATERIALS

In order for your skin care preparations to be effective, they need to be made using high-quality ingredients. If something is selling cheaply, there is usually a reason. For example, some rose fragrances cost about $10 a pound, while certified organic rose costs up to $5,200 a pound (don't worry, you will only need a few drops!). High-quality natural ingredients will always cost more, because the plant from which they came was cultivated without the use of pesticides and often was hand-picked in the wild, both of which processes are very labor intensive. In addition, these very same plants are subject to droughts, weather shifts, insects, and other unpredictable natural forces, making consistent, large yields difficult to achieve. Synthetics are simply easier to handle, which is why most cosmetic houses opt for them. The good news is that a plant or herb that has withstood these conditions is always hardier and possesses more therapeutic value—this is exactly what nature intended: survival of the fittest.

The following pages provide you with details of the basic building blocks and procedures for creating your own skin- and body-care products. Check the Resources section on page 153 for a list of reputable suppliers of essential oils, herbal oils, and natural raw materials.

ESSENTIAL & CARRIER OILS

As a general rule, essential oils need to be diluted and used at low concentrations before you apply them to the skin. The two exceptions to this rule are lavender and tea tree oils, which are gentle enough to be applied neat to the skin.

The way in which essential oils are blended, and the carrier oils or base creams selected will very much depend on the condition you are treating. As a general rule of thumb, when making blends, you will want to use no more than 1 to 2 percent essential oil(s) in the total carrier oil. Products intended for the face will have a lower percentage of essential oil than those intended for the body.

Blending is both an art and a science, and takes practice while you build up familiarity not only with the therapeutic properties of essential oils but also their fragrances. The Aromatherapy Blending Basics section on pages 66–67 will start you on your way. These guidelines will help you decide which essential and carrier oils to use and include tips for how to keep track of the amounts of each oil you selected, for future reference. It may take several tries to get the exact formula that you want; this is the fun part of aromatherapeutic alchemy.

The basic rule for blending is to combine no more than a total of four or five essential oils in a blend. An ideal amount is usually three or four oils; with more than four, the blend begins to get crowded and loses its effectiveness. Select your essential oils in order of therapeutic value. The first will make up the largest percentage of the blend, the second will make up the next largest portion, and so on.

Next, you'll choose a carrier oil. You can select one oil or choose to fortify your blend with a specialty oil such as evening primrose or tamanu oil to boost the therapeutic value of your blend (refer to the Vegetal Oils chart on pages 60–61 to help you decide how much of the oil to use).

Once you have combined your essential and carrier oils and have completed the blend, let the mixture stand for at least 1 hour or up to overnight to let the oils "cook," or amalgamate. You will find that giving the mixture some additional time before using it will allow the oils to open up, creating a more powerful synergistic effect as well as a smoother aromatic bouquet.

Essential oils are light sensitive and should be stored in a cool, dark place in dark-colored bottles. Plastics should never be used, because certain oils are very aggressive and can corrode plastic. Cobalt and amber glass bottles can easily be found at a hardware store or from the specialty aromatherapy suppliers listed in the back of this book.

AROMATHERAPY BLENDING BASICS

Follow these guidelines each time you create a blend. When you begin creating your own blends, it is easy to use too much of one oil or not enough of another. This template helps you to break down that process so you can achieve the optimum results.

Treatment Goal

On a sheet of paper, list what your treatment objectives are—to nourish dry skin, clear up blemishes, reduce scarring, and so on. For example, to treat stress-induced insomnia, the treatment goal might be: Blend a calming nighttime bath oil.

Essential Oils

List the essential oils you've selected and why. You can use a single essential oil or create a blend using no more than a total of five oils. For example, to create the blend in the example above, one possible combination of treatment (essential) oils might be lavender, mandarin, sandalwood, and rose.

Carrier Oils or Lotion

List the carrier oil(s) or lotion you've chosen and why. List the percentage or proportion of each oil used in the blend. For example, for a bath oil, you might want a blend of lightweight oils that will not feel heavy on the skin or leave a tub residue, such as one-third apricot kernel, one-third almond, and one-third sunflower.

Blending Notes

Fill the bottle halfway with the blend of carrier oils. Figure out the total number of drops of essential oils you need using this basic formula: a 4-ounce bottle = total 50 drops, 2-ounce bottle = total 25 drops, 1-ounce bottle = total 12 drops. See the next section for how to determine your blend, but for now, remember that a crucial part of the process is keeping track of the essential oils you include; using hash marks while you count up to each total will help your accuracy. In our example:

CALMING NIGHTTIME BATH OIL
Lavender   ✕✕✕ ✕✕✕ ✕✕✕ |||
Mandarin   ✕✕✕ ✕✕✕ ||||

Total   32 drops
       4-ounce bottle

Blending is both an art and a science and takes practice while you build up familiarity not only with the therapeutic properties of essential oils but also their fragrances.

BLENDING ESSENTIAL OILS

To figure out how many drops of each essential oil to use, begin with your "lead" oil (the one you feel has the greatest therapeutic power to treat the condition) and add what you think is the best number of drops to achieve your goal. Place that number of hash marks next to the name of that oil. Repeat with the remaining oils, screw the cap onto the bottle tightly, and agitate. Open the bottle and smell the oil. If you feel the scent is not quite right, adjust by adding more of a particular oil and document the addition by making the appropriate number of hash marks next to that oil on your list. When the blend seems right, top off the bottle with carrier oil. Agitate a second time.

Use the following as your reference guide in blending essential oils.

Face Serum

Fill a 2-ounce dark-colored glass bottle halfway with a lightweight carrier oil such as apricot kernel, hazelnut, or jojoba. Add 18–24 drops total of essential oil(s). Close the bottle tightly and roll it between your hands to disperse the oils. Open and top off with carrier oil. Recap and agitate a second time.

Massage or Bath Oil

Fill a 4-ounce dark-colored glass bottle halfway with a medium-weight blend of carrier oils that does not feel greasy such as almond, safflower, or sunflower oil. Add 40 to 50 drops total of essential oil(s). Close the bottle tightly and roll it between your hands to disperse the oils. Open and top off with carrier oil. Recap and agitate a second time.

Body Lotion

Fill a 4-ounce bottle one-third full of an unscented lotion or cream made of natural base materials. Add 25 drops total of essential oil(s), close the bottle tightly, and shake well. Open and add another one-third lotion or cream. Add up to 25 more drops essential oil(s), recap, and shake well. Open again and top off to fill with lotion or cream. Recap and agitate a final time.

Herbal Oils, Infusions & Decoctions

Before we move on to the recipes, there is another category of components for creating custom products to add to your arsenal that can add a layer of luxury and lusciousness and healing magic to your final mixes.

Adding herbs to a base or carrier oil can enhance the therapeutic properties of the oil. You can use a solar-infusion technique, using the heat of the sun to gently warm the oil—flowering plants such as arnica, calendula, or St. John's wort are ideal—or a simmering extraction, the preferred method for the leaves of herbs such as rosemary and comfrey, which require more intense heat to pull the active materials from the plant. These oils will keep, tightly sealed in a cool, dark place, for up to 1 year, and can be added to carrier oils or lotions in your formulas.

Extracts can be made from plants using a variety of solvents to pull out the active ingredients. When making herbal infusions, water is used as a solvent and the end product is tea. Herbal infusions can be made with fresh or dried herbs and can be added to creams or balms for the herbs' therapeutic properties.

Herbal decoctions are made by boiling the roots, bark, berries, seeds, and woodier parts of plants in water to extract the active ingredients. This usually requires a longer extraction time than tea due to the nature of the material.

SIMMERED HERBAL OILS

Use this method for making herbal-infused carrier oils when you are working with plant leaves, roots, or any woody material that may be more difficult to extract.

Rosemary Oil

MAKES	1 pint
PREP TIME	2½ hours
YOU WILL NEED	one 1-pint canning jar with lid

A	HR	SR	M

2 cups fresh rosemary leaves

2 cups safflower oil

Cheesecloth or muslin bag

Gently bruise or break the rosemary leaves to extract as much active plant material as possible. Combine the oil and the rosemary in the top pan of a double boiler or a heatproof glass bowl and set over (but not touching) a pan of simmering water. Gently heat the mixture for about 2 hours, then strain through the cheesecloth into the canning jar and screw the lid on tightly. Store in a cool, dark place for 6 to 12 months.

Add the simmered herbal oil to any blend (3 to 10 percent of the total).

SOLAR-INFUSED HERBAL OILS

Solar-infused herbal oils are fun to make in the summer when there is an abundance of fresh plant material and the long, hot days can assist in the production of the oil. In addition to the herbs mentioned above, any number of flowering plants can be used in place of the calendula, such as meadowsweet, lavender, or rose.

Calendula Oil

Research has demonstrated that calendula is beneficial in speeding up wound-healing, making it a valuable herb in repairing the skin barrier. Traditionally, it has been prized for its anti-inflammatory properties. Make this infused herbal oil a staple in your herbal remedy chest for dry skin imbalances.

Calendula *(Calendula officinalis)* **flower heads to fill the jars (2 batches at a 2- to 3-week interval)**

About 2 cups safflower oil

Cheesecloth

MAKES	8 ounces
PREP TIME	About 1 hour, plus about 1 month for the solar infusion
YOU WILL NEED	one 8-ounce dark-colored glass bottle, plus two half-pint canning jars with lids

A   HR   SR   M

Harvest the calendula flowers on a sunny day and discard any soiled parts of the plant. Do not wash the flower heads, since water will encourage mold to grow. Using your hands, gently bruise or break the flowers to extract as much active plant material as possible. Densely pack one of the canning jars to the brim with the flower heads and cover completely with the oil as needed, filling the jar to the rim. Screw the lid on tightly, label with the name of the plant and the date, and leave in a sunny windowsill or greenhouse for 2 to 3 weeks.

Using the cheesecloth, strain the mixture into a measuring cup. Now repeat the process by densely packing the second canning jar with more freshly picked and bruised calendula flower tops and fill to the brim with the reserved once-infused oil. Cover the jar tightly and let steep for 2 to 3 more weeks. Strain the mixture once again through the cheesecloth into an 8-ounce dark-colored glass bottle and store in a cool, dark place for up to 6 to 12 months.

Add the solar-infused herbal oil to any blend (3 to 10 percent of the total).

HERBAL INFUSIONS & DECOCTIONS

Herbs that can be easily used for infusions include green tea, rosemary, borage, calendula, chamomile, lemon balm, geranium, and rose petals. Use herbal infusions to make toners or balms, or add to bath water to enhance the therapeutic effect of the bath.

Herbal decoctions can also be used to supplement balms, or can be added to bath water to enhance the therapeutic effect of the bath. Plants that can be extracted with herbal decoctions include burdock root, dandelion root, echinacea root, and schisandra berry, to name a few.

Basic Herbal Infusion

MAKES	1 cup
PREP TIME	15 minutes
YOU WILL NEED	one half-pint canning jar with lid

A HR SR M

2 ounces fresh herbs, bruised, or 1 ounce dried

1 cup distilled water

Cheesecloth

Place the herbs in a French press. In a small saucepan, bring the distilled water to a boil over high heat. Pour the hot water over the herbs. Let steep for 10 minutes. Strain the tea through the cheesecloth into the canning jar. Add this mixture directly to toners or balms or add herbal infusions to bath water and discard any leftover infusion.

Basic Herbal Decoction

MAKES	3 cups
PREP TIME	45 minutes
YOU WILL NEED	one 1-quart canning jar with lid

A HR SR M

1 ounce fresh herbs, bruised, or ½ ounce dried

4 cups distilled water

Cheesecloth

Break up the plant material by chopping with a knife or crushing it in a mortar using a pestle. Place the herbs and distilled water in a saucepan, bring the water to a boil, and simmer until the liquid is reduced to about 3 cups, about 15 minutes. Cover and let steep for an additional 10 minutes. Strain through the cheesecloth into the canning jar and let cool. Cover tightly and store in the refrigerator for up to 4 days.

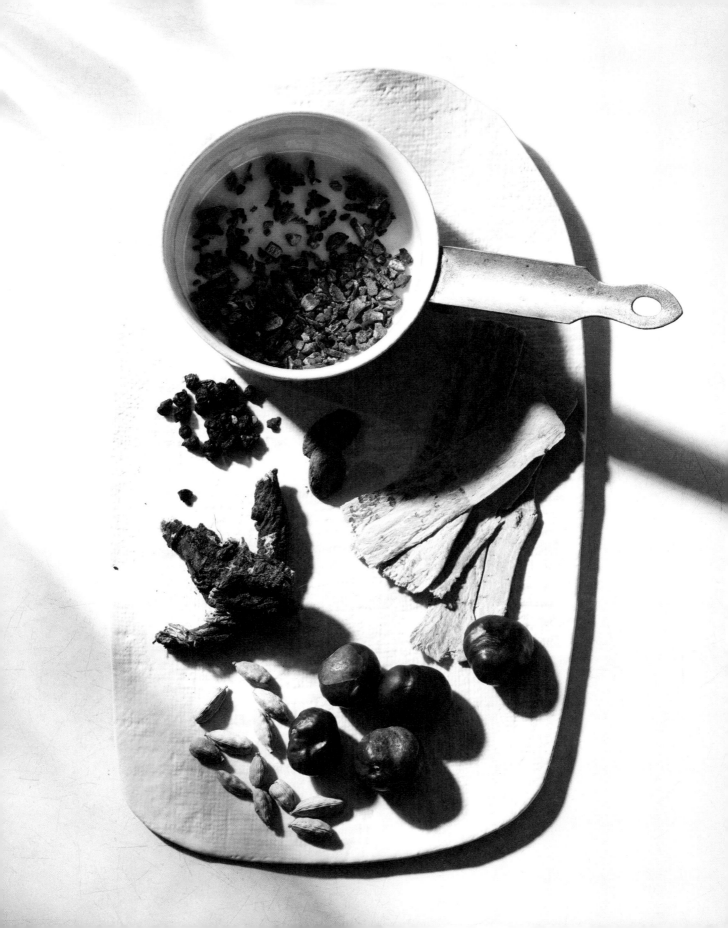

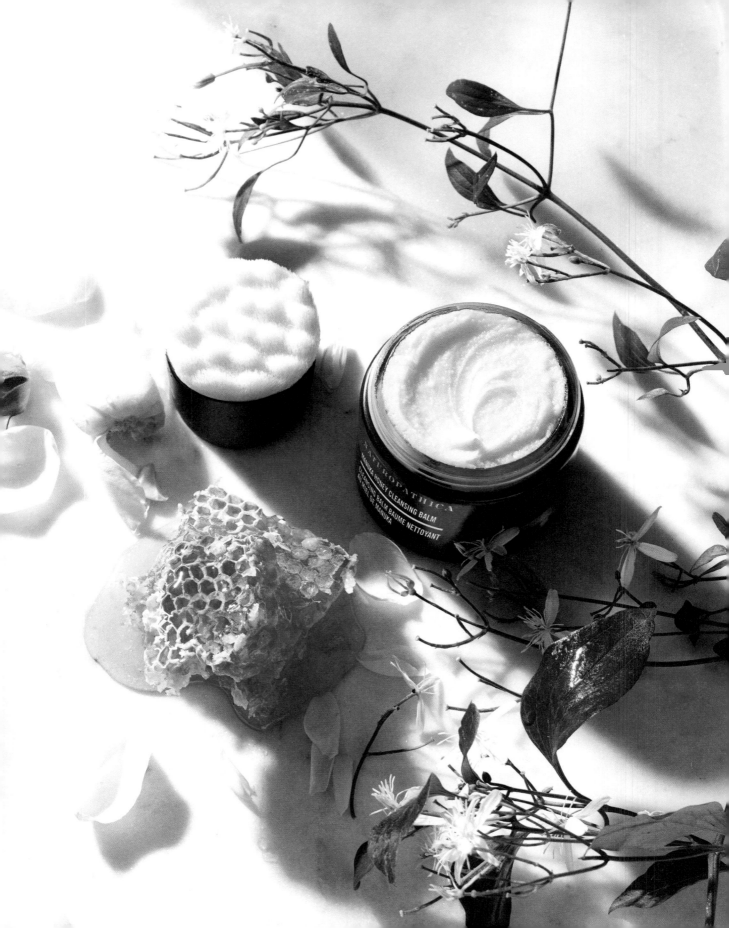

The Recipes

Now that you know the basics of holistic skin care, you're ready to try making some of your own all-natural skin care products. The essential oils and herbal derivatives described in the previous section form the building blocks for cleansers and moisturizers for the face and body.

CLEANSERS

Cleansing is the most important step of your skin care regimen, so you want to be sure you are not using an aggressive surfactant that is stripping the good oils from your skin and thus promoting irritation. Most skin imbalances are caused by over-cleansing of the skin, since we have been conditioned to believe that only harsh, foamy cleansers are effective. This creates a whole host of problems as the skin tries to correct itself.

Gently removing dirt and product buildup while strengthening the skin barrier is the essence of a good cleansing regimen. Nature provides excellent alternatives to synthetic commercial cleansers, with antiseptic essential oils and organic base materials that respect the integrity of the skin.

Clarifying Cleansing Oil

This cleansing oil has antiseptic essential oils in it to eliminate blackheads. The light, vegetal oil base contains jojoba oil, similar to our skin's own sebum, and will not clog pores. Rosemary essential oil is rich in antioxidants.

1½ ounces apricot kernel oil

12 drops rosemary *(Rosmarinus officinalis)* essential oil

6 drops lavender *(Lavandula vera)* essential oil

4 drops cypress *(Cupressus sempervirens)* essential oil

½ ounce jojoba oil

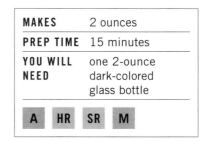

MAKES	2 ounces
PREP TIME	15 minutes
YOU WILL NEED	one 2-ounce dark-colored glass bottle

A HR SR M

Pour the apricot kernel oil into the bottle. Add the essential oils, close the bottle tightly, and roll it between your palms to disperse the oils. Open and top off with the jojoba oil. Close the bottle tightly again and agitate a second time.

Rinse your face with warm water. Apply a small amount of the cleansing oil to the pads of your fingers or a cotton pad and wipe over your face and throat area, gently loosening any makeup or grime. Place a hot towel over your face. When the towel has cooled down, gently wipe your face with the towel until all of the oil residue is removed.

Cleansing Facial Gommage

MAKES	½ cup
PREP TIME	30 minutes

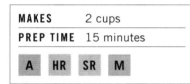

Gommage means "to erase" in French, and here refers to the process of exfoliating the skin and removing dead skin cells. This scrub is easy to prepare and will leave your skin smooth and polished. Oats contain oat beta glucan, which forms a film to help the skin retain moisture and also has anti-inflammatory properties to help soothe aggravated skin.

¼ cup Basic Herbal Infusion (page 70) made with chamomile or calendula

¼ cup rolled oats

1 tablespoon honey

Prepare the herbal infusion and set aside to steep. Meanwhile, in a blender, grind the oats into a coarse (not fine) flour. Transfer to a bowl and stir in the honey. Pour the ¼ cup herbal infusion over the oat mixture, stir to combine well, and set aside for 5 minutes.

Rinse your face with warm water. Apply a small amount of the gommage to the pads of your fingers and gently massage all over your face, taking care not to overstimulate the skin by scrubbing too long. Discard any leftover gommage.

Clarifying Facial Sauna

MAKES	2 cups
PREP TIME	15 minutes

Contrary to popular belief, a facial steam bath does not open pores. Pores do not fluctuate in size, but they do fill up with dirt and debris. A good facial steam with antiseptic and stimulating essential oils and herbs helps to promote circulation and soften the skin, making the process of removing impurities easier.

1 ounce fresh rosemary leaves, bruised

1 ounce fresh basil leaves, bruised

1 sprig fresh thyme, bruised

2 cups distilled water

4 drops lavender *(Lavandula vera)* essential oil

Combine all of the herbs in a French press. In a small saucepan, bring the distilled water to a rolling boil. Pour the boiling water over the herbs and let steep for 10 minutes. Meanwhile, keep the tea kettle going with hot water to add extra heat to your facial steam.

Fill a clean bathroom sink with hot tap water. Add the lavender essential oil to the water and swish with your hand to disperse the oil. Strain the herbal infusion from the French press into the water in the sink. Cover your head and shoulders with a towel and lean over the basin, making a tent with the towel to hold in the steam. Allow skin to soften in warm, humid air for 5 minutes while inhaling relaxing aromas, adding more hot water from the kettle as needed.

TONERS

Toners not only help adjust the pH level of your skin, they can also help remove any traces of dirt left after cleansing. The best toners are hydrolats, also called floral waters, which are by-products of the steam distillation process used to extract essential oils. When plant material, such as lavender, is exposed to steam, volatile therapeutic compounds are released into the water. The essential oil is then drawn off, leaving the hydrosol, which contains molecules of essential oils and constituents of the herb or flower. Like homeopathic medicines, these waters possess a vibrational energy that can be used to help balance and fortify the skin.

In the following recipes, essential oils are added to distilled water in order to nourish and balance the skin. Herbal teas also make good base materials for toners and are easy to prepare. For more astringency, add apple cider vinegar.

Green Tea Toner

Green tea is well known for its antioxidant properties, and aloe vera acts as a humectant to draw moisture into the skin. Use this toner after cleansing to recharge your skin and make it glow.

4 teaspoons green tea leaves

1 teaspoon dried peppermint leaves

4 ounces distilled water

2 drops lavender *(Lavandula vera)* essential oil

2 teaspoons aloe vera gel

MAKES	4 ounces
PREP TIME	15 minutes
YOU WILL NEED	one 4-ounce dark-colored glass bottle with spray atomizer

A HR SR M

Combine the herbs in a French press. In a small saucepan, bring the distilled water to a rolling boil. Pour the boiling water over the herbs. Add the lavender essential oil and let steep for 10 minutes, then plunge and let cool. Pour the aloe vera gel into the bottle and fill with the herbal infusion. Cap with the spray atomizer and shake well.

Spritz your face liberally. Store the toner in the refrigerator for up to 30 days.

Clarifying Parsley Toner

MAKES	4 ounces
PREP TIME	20 minutes
YOU WILL NEED	one 4-ounce dark-colored glass bottle with spray atomizer

HR

This toner is excellent for skin that is hormone reactive (see pages 36–37) or prone to breakouts and blemishes. Parsley is a clarifying herb and tea tree oil has strong antiseptic properties that help clear up blemishes. Apple cider vinegar is also an important blemish fighter because it has a high acid content and the bacteria causing blemishes cannot thrive in such an acidic environment.

1 ounce fresh parsley leaves, bruised

½ cup distilled water

1 tablespoon apple cider vinegar

4 drops tea tree oil

Put the parsley in a French press. In a small saucepan, bring the distilled water to a rolling boil. Pour the boiling water over the parsley. Let steep for 10 minutes, then plunge and let cool. Pour the apple cider vinegar and the tea tree oil into the bottle and fill with the parsley infusion. Cap with the spray atomizer and shake well.

Spritz your face liberally. Store the toner in the refrigerator for up to 30 days.

Plant Milk

MAKES	4 ounces
PREP TIME	20 minutes
YOU WILL NEED	one 4-ounce dark-colored glass bottle with spray atomizer

SR

This recipe is wonderful in the wintertime when your skin is feeling raw or exposed, or anytime your skin feels dry or sensitive. This "plant milk" is derived from oats, a natural skin soother, and also contains calendula, a traditional anti-inflammatory herb. It will leave the skin feeling soft and moisturized.

1 ounce dried calendula flowers

½ cup rolled oats

12 ounces distilled water

Combine the flowers and oats in a French press. In a small saucepan, bring the distilled water to a rolling boil. Pour the boiling water over the flowers and oats. Let steep for 10 minutes, then plunge and let cool. Pour the infusion into the bottle, cap with the spray atomizer, and shake well.

Spritz your face liberally. Store the toner in the refrigerator for up to 30 days.

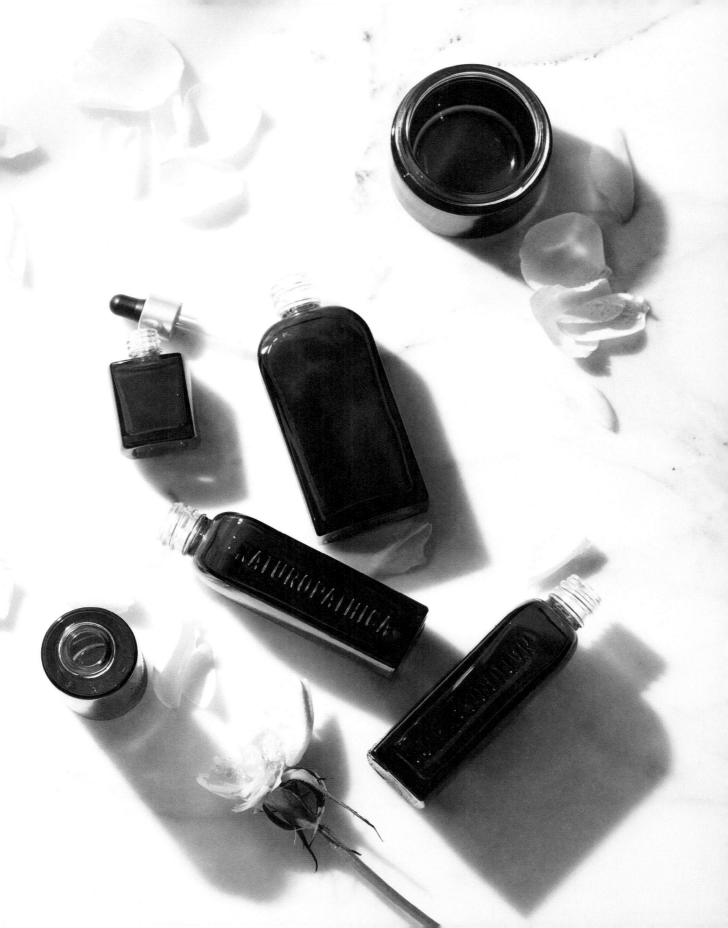

MOISTURIZERS & FACIAL OILS

All moisturizers are simply an emulsion of oil and water. The purpose is twofold: to draw moisture into the skin and seal it in (this is why it is always a good idea to put on a moisturizer right after you have cleaned your face, while the skin is still damp); and to nourish and support the outer layers of the skin by filling up the gaps between the layers of the cells.

You can buy all-natural base creams and lotions from a natural skin care supplier (see Resources, page 153). I don't recommend making creams at home, as it is not possible to achieve the smooth texture of a professionally made natural cream, and because homemade creams will need to be refrigerated. Alternatively, facial oils are easy to prepare at home and deliver the results you need. Think of facial oils as your custom-blended skin conditioners.

Neroli Toning Facial Oil

MAKES	2 ounces
PREP TIME	20 minutes
YOU WILL NEED	one 2-ounce dark-colored glass bottle
A	

The blossoming flowers of neroli and ylang-ylang give this serum its rich, luxurious scent. Adding the antiseptic properties of thyme and the skin-cell-regenerating abilities of rosemary produces a mix that's an ideal daily maintenance oil for balanced skin.

1 ounce hazelnut oil or apricot kernel oil

6 drops neroli (Citrus aurantium) essential oil

5 drops ylang-ylang (Cananga odorata) essential oil

4 drops rosemary (Rosmarinus officinalis) essential oil

2 drops thyme (Thymus vulgaris, linalool type) essential oil

1 ounce jojoba oil

Pour the hazelnut oil into the bottle. Add the essential oils, close the bottle tightly, and roll it between your palms to disperse the oils. Open and top off with the jojoba oil. Close the bottle tightly again and agitate a second time.

To cleanse and tone the skin, apply 3 or 4 drops of the facial oil to a cotton pad or the pads of your fingers and smooth over your entire face. For enhanced results, use the serum in conjunction with a Facial Massage (page 81).

Carrot Seed Protective Facial Oil

This serum is beneficial for calming and nourishing dry or sensitive skin. The combination of soothing vegetal oils, argan, avocado, and evening primrose revitalizes dull skin with a high concentration of vitamins and essential fatty acids. The regenerating and stimulating properties of carrot seed and rosemary essential oils help to bring the skin back to life.

MAKES	2 ounces
PREP TIME	20 minutes
YOU WILL NEED	one 2-ounce dark-colored glass bottle
SR	

1 ounce argan oil

6 drops rose *(Rosa damascena)* essential oil

5 drops carrot seed *(Daucus carota)* essential oil

4 drops lavender *(Lavandula vera)* essential oil

3 drops geranium oil *(Pelargonium graveolens)* essential oil

½ ounce avocado oil

½ ounce evening primrose oil

Pour the argan oil into the bottle. Add the essential oils, close the bottle tightly, and roll it between your palms to disperse the oils. Open and top off with the avocado and evening primrose oils. Close the bottle tightly again and agitate a second time.

To cleanse and tone the skin, apply 3 or 4 drops of the facial oil to a cotton pad or the pads of your fingers and smooth over your entire face. For enhanced results, use the serum in conjunction with a Facial Massage (page 81).

Blemish Facial Oil

The two base oils used in this recipe, hazelnut and apricot kernel, are two of the lightest weight, most astringent oils. Tea tree oil helps to break down hardened sebum and is well known for its strong antibacterial qualities. Rosemary, a strong skin-cell-regenerating oil, combines nicely with the tonifying properties of lavender and juniper.

MAKES	2 ounces
PREP TIME	20 minutes
YOU WILL NEED	one 2-ounce dark-colored glass bottle
HR	

1 ounce marula oil

8 drops rosemary *(Rosmarinus officinalis)* essential oil

6 drops Lavender *(Lavandula vera)* essential oil

5 drops juniper *(Juniperus communis)* essential oil

5 drops tea tree *(Melaleuca alternifolia)* essential oil

1 ounce apricot kernel oil

Pour the marula oil into the bottle. Add the essential oils, close the bottle tightly, and roll it between your palms to disperse the oils. Open and top off with the apricot kernel oil. Close the bottle tightly again and agitate a second time.

To cleanse and tone skin, apply 3 or 4 drops of the facial oil to a cotton pad or the pads of your fingers and smooth over your entire face. For enhanced results, use the serum in conjunction with a Facial Massage (page 81).

Geranium Regenerating Facial Oil

MAKES	2 ounces
PREP TIME	20 minutes
YOU WILL NEED	one 2-ounce dark-colored glass bottle

M

Mature skin is thinner than the skin of younger people and often lacks sufficient moisture. The combination of vegetal oils in this serum results in the highest possible percentage of GLA, an essential fatty acid in collagen synthesis that makes the skin firmer (see page 59). The geranium aroma provides a lovely sumptuousness, but the real heart of this serum is the everlasting essential oil. Also called *immortelle*, everlasting earns its reputation by keeping skin looking younger. A potent anti-inflammatory herb, it helps remedy broken capillaries, soothes dry skin, and assists in cellular repair.

1 ounce baobab oil

7 drops frankincense *(Boswellia carteri)* essential oil

6 drops everlasting *(Helichrysum italicum)* essential oil

5 drops geranium *(Pelargonium odoratissimum)* essential oil

2 drops chamomile *(Matricaria reticulata)* essential oil

⅓ ounce rose hip seed oil

⅓ ounce evening primrose oil

⅓ ounce avocado oil

Pour the baobab oil into the bottle. Add the essential oils, close the bottle tightly, and roll it between your palms to disperse the oils. Open and top off with the rose hip seed oil, evening primrose oil, and avocado oil. Close the bottle tightly again and agitate a second time.

To cleanse and tone your skin, apply 3 or 4 drops of the facial oil to a cotton pad or the pads of your fingers and smooth over your entire face. For enhanced results (to plump up the skin), use the facial oil in conjunction with a facial massage (right).

FACIAL MASSAGE

Facial massage benefits the skin in many ways. First, it stimulates blood circulation to the tissues, increasing the supply of nutrients and oxygen. Second, the increased circulatory flow creates heat, which allows the essential oils to penetrate the skin more easily. Massage also relaxes the superficial and deep facial muscles, of which there are over thirty. When these muscles become tight, they constrict the blood flow and the supply of vital nutrients that feed the skin.

To give yourself a facial massage, start with a lavender compress. Compresses are relaxing moist-heat treatments that increase local circulation to improve dull facial complexions. Fill your bathroom sink with warm water. Add 2 or 3 drops of lavender (*Lavandula vera*) essential oil and swish the water to disperse the oil. Soak a washcloth in the oiled water, wring out, and apply to your face. Inhale deeply to receive the relaxing benefits.

Apply a facial oil (see page 78) to the pads of your fingers and rub your hands together to warm the oil. Gently press the oil onto your face, beginning at the chin and working up towards your hairline, using small, circular movements. At the center of your forehead, sweep your fingertips out towards your temples. Repeat the same circular strokes beginning on either side of the nose and moving laterally to massage your cheeks, jawline, and chin. Follow by stimulating your facial reflex points (right) to increase energy flow.

FACIAL REFLEX POINTS

Press and hold each point for 5 seconds, using medium pressure:

1 Using your thumb, press down at the supraorbital notch at the inside of each eyebrow on either side of your nose. Finish by gliding your thumbs outward across your eyebrows.

2 Using your index fingers, press down at the outside edge of each eyebrow.

3 Using your index fingers, press down on either side of the nose, below the orbital bone just below the pupil of each eye.

4 Using your index fingers, repeat ¼ inch below the last reflex points on either side of your nose.

5 Repeat again, ¼ inch below the last reflex point on either side of your nose.

6 Using your index fingers, gently press on the TMJ (temporomandibular) joints of your jaw, the hinge joints that allow your mouth to open and close.

7 Finish the treatment with a second lavender compress to increase the absorption of the essential oils.

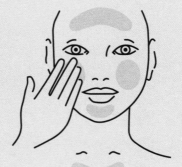

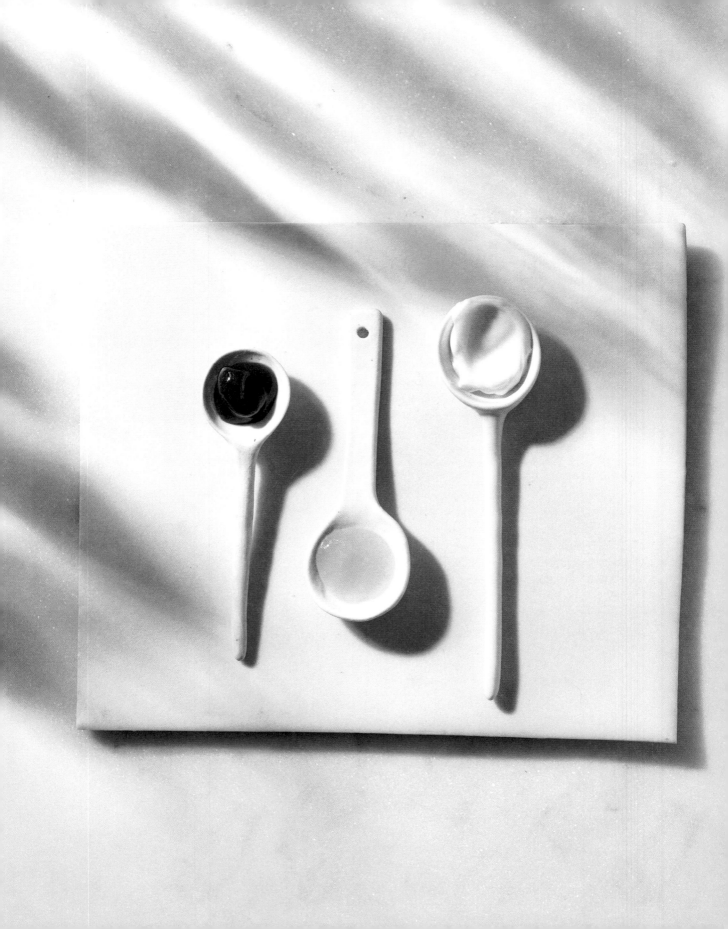

MASKS

The purpose of a mask is to recharge your skin, either by adding more moisture, exfoliating dead skin cells, or clearing away excess oil. Applying a mask is also a good opportunity to give the skin a dose of vitamins, antioxidants, and essential fatty acids, especially if you have been on the go and haven't been maintaining a proper skin care regimen.

Avocado Matcha Mask

There is a reason every skin care book has a recipe for an avocado mask: this fruit is simply so rich in proteins, vitamins, lecithin, and essential fatty acids, it's like a well-balanced meal for the skin.

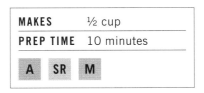

MAKES	½ cup
PREP TIME	10 minutes

A SR M

1 ripe avocado, peeled and pitted

1 egg

1 tablespoon plain yogurt

1 teaspoon baking soda

¼ teaspoon matcha green tea powder

2 drops chamomile *(Matricaria recutita)* essential oil

1 drop lavender *(Lavandula vera)* essential oil

1 tablespoon coconut oil (optional)

Combine all the ingredients in a blender and process until smooth, about 30 seconds. Apply immediately to clean skin and leave on for 5 to 10 minutes. Rinse off with warm water.

Purifying Green Tea Mask

Clays are traditionally used in skin care for their drying properties; as they dry, they pull out excess oil and dirt and leave the skin feeling clean. This mask uses kaolin and bentonite clays, which are sold at health-food and specialty stores and online.

MAKES	¼ cup
PREP TIME	10 minutes

HR

1 tablespoon Basic Herbal Infusion (page 70) made with green tea

2 teaspoons aloe vera gel

1 teaspoon honey

2 tablespoons kaolin clay

1 tablespoon bentonite clay

2 drops rosemary *(Rosmarinus officinalis)* essential oil

2 drops lavender *(Lavandula vera)* essential oil

Combine the green tea infusion, aloe vera gel, and honey in a bowl and stir well. Slowly sprinkle in the kaolin and bentonite clays while stirring. Add the essential oils and stir to combine well. Apply to your clean face immediately and leave on for 10 minutes. Rinse off with warm water.

HAND CARE

The hands are fascinating appendages—small peninsulas of flesh and bone that are our loyal servants, carrying out our most basic needs and desires: dialing a phone number, opening a door, eating an apple, or caressing a lover. If you are like me, your hands also receive a fair amount of abuse. They fidget and wring, pull weeds, wash dishes, and do hundreds of other tasks. Add to that exposure to the elements, and our hands may not be a very pretty sight.

The good news is that there are a lot of nourishing rituals and recipes for the hands, which are usually very forgiving when treated properly.

Hand Soak

MAKES	about 2 cups
PREP TIME	45 minutes

A   HR   SR   M

Begin your repentance by doing a hand soak.

2 cups warm water

1 tablespoon milk

1 teaspoon baking soda

3 drops tea tree *(Melaleuca alternifolia)* essential oil (optional)

2 tablespoons white wine vinegar (optional)

1 tablespoon fresh lemon juice (optional)

Put the warm water in a bowl and stir in the milk and baking soda. Soak your hands in the warm mixture for 5 minutes to soften your cuticles. If your cuticles are ragged and sore, add the tea tree oil to facilitate the healing process.

Remove your hands from the bath and dry them. Clip and file your nails and push back any cuticles that are in need of maintenance. If any of your nails are discolored, soak them again, but this time add the white wine vinegar and lemon juice.

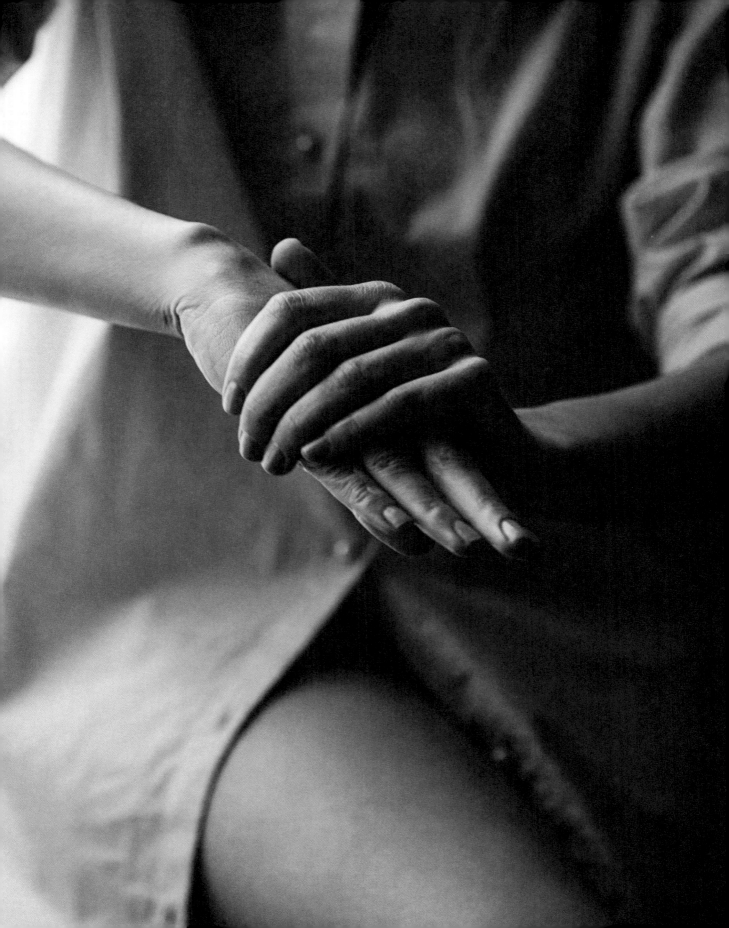

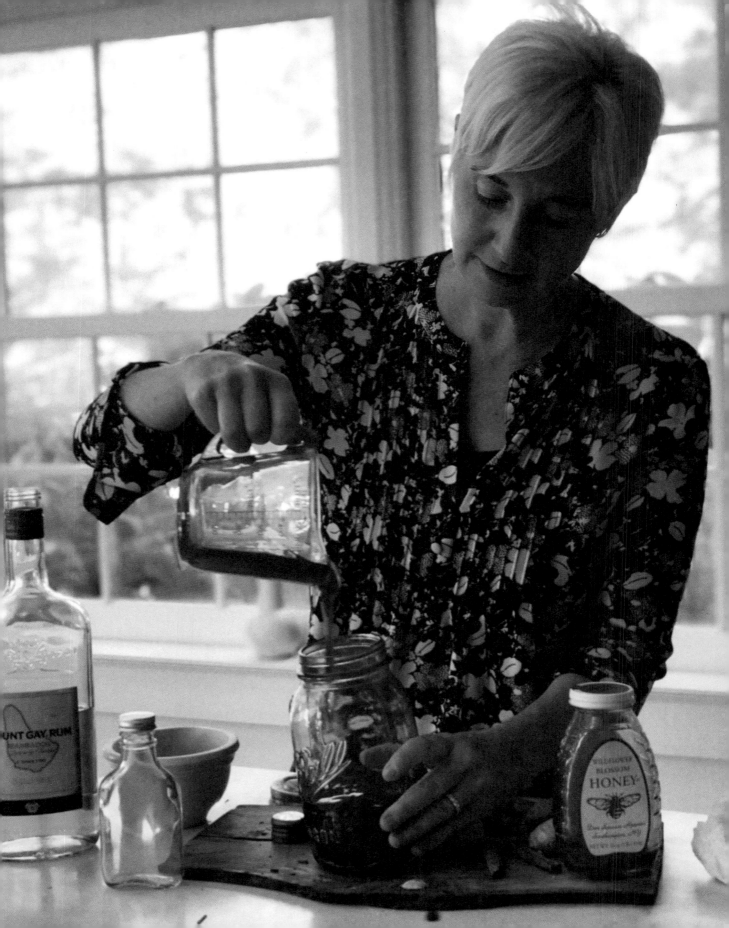

Whipped Shea Butter Hand Softener

This luxurious softener for hands going through a rough period is fortified with rich avocado oil and whipped with creamy cocoa and shea butters to deeply penetrate the skin so there is no greasy film. The fresh, uplifting neroli flower scent is hypnotic.

MAKES	6 ounces
PREP TIME	45 minutes
YOU WILL NEED	one 6-ounce dark-colored glass jar with lid

| A | HR | SR | M |

2 ounces avocado oil

2 ounces cocoa butter

1 ounce beeswax

1 ounce shea butter

8 drops neroli *(Citrus aurantium)* essential oil

3 drops sandalwood *(Santalum album)*

Place the glass jar in a saucepan filled with water and gently boil for 5 minutes to sterilize the jar.

Meanwhile, melt the avocado oil, cocoa butter, and beeswax together in the top pan of a double boiler or a heatproof bowl set over (but not touching) a pan of simmering water. Add the shea butter and immediately remove from the heat. Stir until all the chunks of cocoa and shea butter are completely melted. Add the neroli and sandalwood essential oils and stir again to mix well.

Place the bowl in the freezer until the top layer solidifies. Remove the bowl from the freezer. Using an immersion blender, whip the mixture until a butter-like consistency is achieved. Transfer to the jar. Cover tightly and store for up to 12 months.

FOOT CARE

There are over 250,000 sweat glands in the soles of the feet. So, when confined to the airtight humidors of our shoes all day, it's no wonder our feet look the way they do. These next recipes provide a little TLC for your hardworking feet.

Nail Fungus Relief

MAKES	1 Tablespoon
PREP TIME	20 minutes
YOU WILL NEED	one ½-ounce dark-colored glass bottle

A	HR	SR	M

Here is an effective remedy for that unsightly yellow nail fungus—although tea tree oil, the standard cure-all for nail fungus, may not be strong enough if the fungus has been allowed to grow unhindered for some time. This recipe combines the powerful antiseptic action of three phenol-type essential oils: thyme, tea tree, and oregano.

1 tablespoon sunflower oil

30 drops thyme *(Thymus vulgaris, thymol type)* essential oil

15 drops oregano *(Origanum vulgaris)* essential oil

15 drops tea tree *(Melaleuca alternifolia)* essential oil

Pour half of the sunflower oil into the bottle. Add the essential oils, close the bottle tightly, and shake well. Top off with the remaining sunflower oil, close the bottle tightly again, and agitate a second time. Apply to affected areas twice a day. Discontinue use after 1 month if you see no signs of improvement.

Peppermint Foot Bath

MAKES	1 Tablespoon
PREP TIME	20 minutes

A	HR	SR	M

The restorative hot foot bath is a popular naturopathic technique that draws blood away from the head and extremities in order to release toxins and ease stress. (This same technique is an effective natural remedy for getting rid of headaches by drawing excess blood from the head to the feet.)

1 Tablespoon sunflower oil

3 drops peppermint *(Mentha piperita)* essential oil

Fill a large bowl or small tub with hot water. Combine the sunflower oil and peppermint essential oil and add to the water. Swish with your hand to disperse the oil. Place your feet in the bath and soak for 5 to 10 minutes, until your feet feel cool and tingly. For extra stimulation, place some pebbles or marbles in the tub and roll your feet back and forth over them.

Rosemary-Peppermint Foot Scrub

Remove dry, calloused skin with this stimulating exfoliating paste.

MAKES	½ cup
PREP TIME	10 minutes

A	HR	SR	M

1 tablespoon sunflower oil

3 drops rosemary *(Rosmarinus officinalis)* essential oil

3 drops peppermint *(Mentha piperita)* essential oil

½ cup stone-ground cornmeal

In a bowl, combine the sunflower oil with the rosemary and peppermint essential oils. Slowly stir in the cornmeal until a thick paste forms. Apply the mixture to the soles of your feet in a circular scrubbing motion, paying special attention to callous-prone heels and toes.

NOTE For deeper exfoliation of extra-calloused feet, use sea salt instead of cornmeal.

Tea Tree and Lemon Foot Balm

Antiseptic tea tree and lemon essential oils blend together beautifully in this recipe to revitalize tired feet.

MAKES	2 ounces
PREP TIME	45 minutes
YOU WILL NEED	one 2-ounce dark-colored glass jar

A	HR	SR	M

3 tablespoons shea butter

1 tablespoon coconut oil

1 tablespoon Basic Herbal Infusion (page 70) made with lemon balm

5 drops lemon *(Citrus limonum)* essential oil

3 drops tea tree *(Melaleuca alternifolia)* essential oil

Place the jar in a saucepan filled with water and gently boil for 5 minutes to sterilize the jar. Meanwhile, melt the shea butter and coconut oil together in the top pan of a double boiler or a heatproof glass measuring cup in a shallow pan of simmering water and stir with a spoon to mix thoroughly. Add the lemon balm infusion and essential oils and mix into a smooth cream. Dispense into the jar and use for foot massage (see page 129). Keep refrigerated to discourage spoiling.

Chapter 4

The Beauty Kitchen

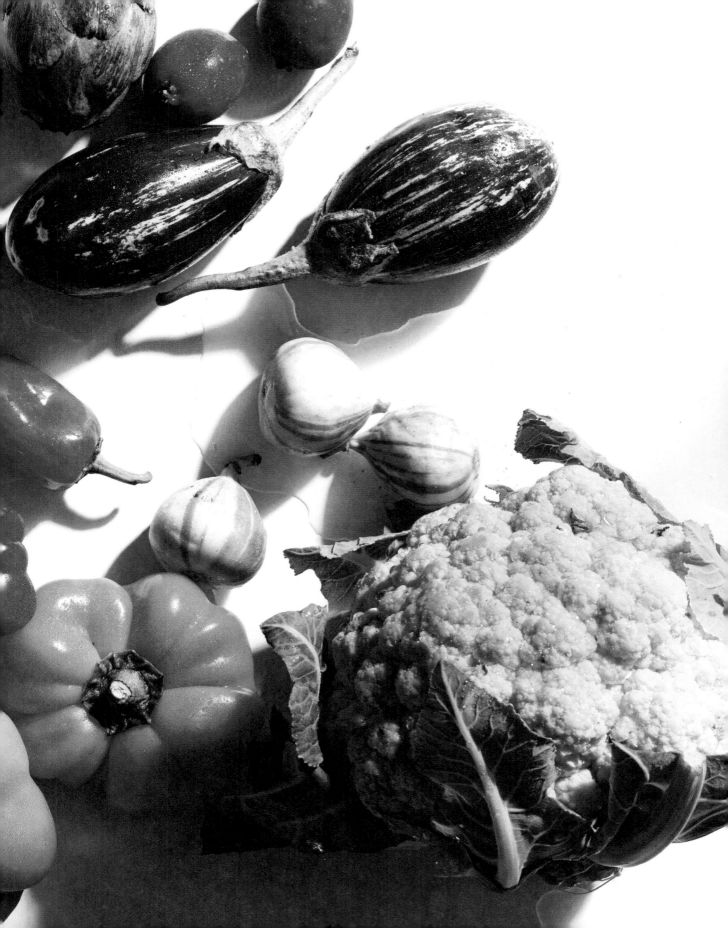

W e all have our own unique relationship to eating. For me, I have come to forgive my excesses and, in fact, accept them if I can fit them into a larger context of eating healthier. My credo, "Everything in moderation—even moderation," speaks to the inevitability of eating cassoulet or an apple-butterscotch tart, but within the broader context of knowing how to balance those indulgences with healthy food staples and healthy eating habits. My aim in this chapter is to share some of these health-sustaining tips.

Eating Well

As the crusade against smoking continues to mount a successful campaign, the next public health issue to come under scrutiny is food. Recently released government data shows that more than one-third of children and two out of three adults are considered overweight or obese.[1] The problem is not only the quantity of food Americans are eating, but also the quality of the food, primarily convenience foods. These empty foods, loaded with sugar, refined flour, genetically modified grains, hydrogenated fats, additives, and preservatives wreak havoc on our bodies. To make matters worse, modern industrial farming has depleted our soil, yielding fruits and vegetables with far fewer vitamins and minerals and making it more difficult to get the nutrients our body needs.

The essence of the Slow Food movement is to take the time to enjoy locally grown food and ingredients as opposed to grabbing a panini at a fast-food restaurant. Think of a dinner with roasted free-range chicken, vegetables in season from a local farm, and a glass of wine from a nearby vineyard. In my opinion, it doesn't get better than this. But agribusiness wants to get a uniform food product to your table as fast as possible. This means using a lot of pesticides as well as genetically engineered, pest-resistant seeds in order to cultivate soil that yields more per acre at the expense of nutrients and taste. If you have had a hard time recently finding a tomato or an ear of corn that actually tastes good, you've experienced the outcome of this process.

For the best skin-nourishing nutrients, choose organic foods whenever you can. In addition to their lack of potentially carcinogenic pesticides, organic foods have been shown to be higher in nutrients than conventionally grown foods. Anyone who has ever tended a garden can attest to the vibrancy and lushness of a just-picked cantaloupe or tomato. Fresh, organically grown plant material has a vibrational energy that nourishes the body right down to the cellular level. The hydrogenated, indefinitely preserved, prepackaged food that we see at our supermarket has almost none of the vitamins, nutrients, or vitality of the plant material from which it came.

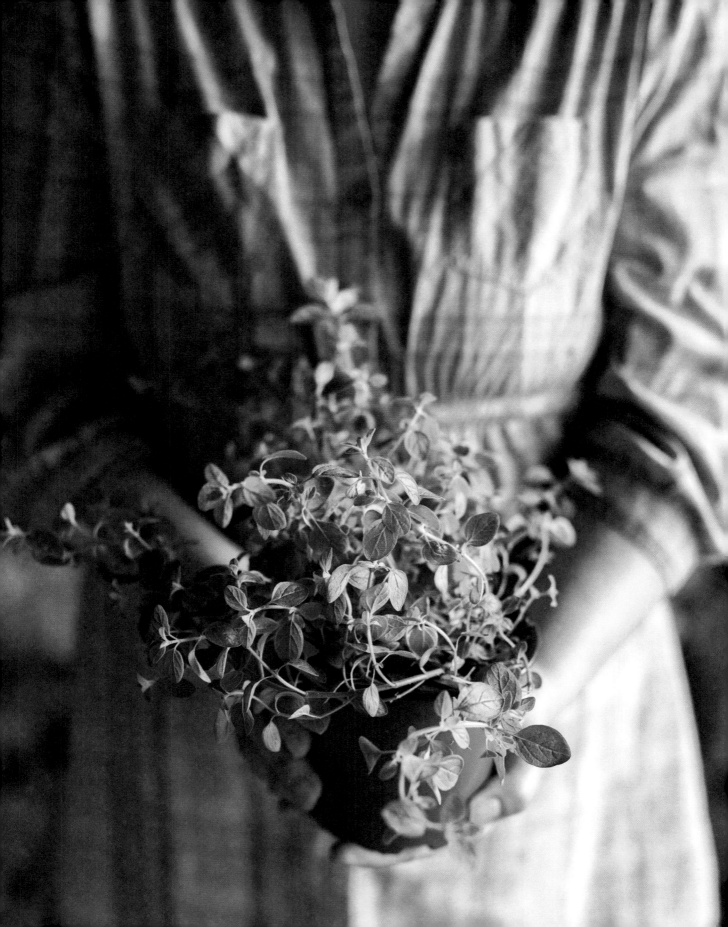

Studies published over the last fifteen years show that due to nonsustainable farming practices, many of our vegetables have dropped in key nutrients that prevent disease, such as vitamins, minerals, and phytonutrients—up to 30 percent less in the case of vitamin C and 27 percent less in calcium levels.[2]

One solution is to forage, since many plants in the wild, for example field garlic, chickweed, watercress, and those prolific dandelion leaves, are rich in polyphenols, protective antioxidants. Urban dwellers might look for arugula at the supermarket when making salads instead of lettuce; this plant has retained many of its wild ancestral roots and is rich in antioxidants as well as glucosinolates, a key liver detoxifier. Scallions remain quite similar to their wild onion cousins and are also a good source of phytonutrients (especially the green parts). But simple awareness is a great asset—just adding a couple of tablespoons of fresh, organic herbs—basil, parsley, thyme, oregano, rosemary, or mint—will help bring back phytonutrients to your daily allowance.

DESTRUCTIVE FOODS

There are some foods whose effects on the body make us feel bad physiologically as well as emotionally, by triggering cravings and profound chemical changes in the body. The most destructive of these changes in terms of skin care is the inflammatory response that the body develops to combat irritants. To prevent this inflammatory response, stick to low-glycemic foods. These are foods that do not rapidly convert to sugar, the most destructive inflammatory agent. High-glycemic foods include pasta, desserts, candy, and even high-starch vegetables like potatoes and corn. One of the most misleading beauty myths is cold-pressed juices. Although they possess lots of vitamins and minerals, they have less fiber and spike blood-sugar levels. To learn more about what foods are high on the glycemic index, visit www.glycemicindex.com.

My advice is to know thy enemy: indulge in the foods discussed below if you must, but make it the exception, not the rule.

Sugar

Sugar causes inflammation in several ways. When blood sugar goes up, it creates free radicals that attack our body on a cellular level by oxidizing fats. These oxidized fats convert to chemical compounds called aldehydes that trigger an inflammatory response. Sugar is bad for just about every system in the body, such as the immune system, the cardiovascular system (it raises HDL, the bad cholesterol), and especially the skin, as it breaks down the lipid barriers of the cells. Sugar also encourages glycation and wrinkles by causing collagen and elastin to become stiff and rigid. Try an herbal remedy called stevia, available in health-food stores, to sweeten your beverages naturally. Stevia is three hundred times stronger than sugar but does not have the harmful inflammatory side effects.

Refined Flour

Refined flours, such as the all-purpose white flour used for many pastas and breads, are also high-glycemic starches that act like sugars. Whole grains, on the other hand, contain health-enhancing bran (the outer layer) and germ (the internal seed) naturally found in all grains, which have fiber as well as nutritive phytochemicals. Several studies have documented that people with diets that include whole grains, as opposed to refined flour, live longer.[3] My favorite grain is quinoa, a gluten-free grain with a high protein and amino-acid content. Other gluten-free options are brown rice, amaranth, and buckwheat.

Hydrogenated Fats

Also known as trans-fatty acids, hydrogenated fats are common in many fast-food and packaged goods to extend their shelf life. These fats wreak havoc on the body by unleashing free radicals that play a role in heart disease and cancer, and have a strong inflammatory response in the body.

Acid-Forming Foods

Acid-forming foods such as coffee, alcohol, processed foods, and saturated fats from dairy and red meat can aggravate skin disturbances. Eat a more alkaline diet of grains, fruits, and vegetables, especially if you are a Hormone Reactive or Stress Reactive skin personality (see pages 36 and 40). If you feel like you are eating carefully but your skin is persistently itching or is prone to rashes and other irritations, I recommend buying a pH kit from a health-food store. These kits are easy to use and will demonstrate the acid or alkalinity in your body based on a saliva test.

FOOD SENSITIVITIES

Many people have food sensitivities to common foods such as wheat (and gluten), corn, soybeans, nuts, eggs, dairy, or nightshade fruits and vegetables (tomatoes, potatoes, peppers, eggplant). A food sensitivity is an immune-system response to a food that our body perceives as harmful. Common signs of food sensitivities are skin rashes, dark circles under the eyes, bloating, excess mucus, and muscle aches. Removing problem foods from your diet can dramatically improve chronic skin conditions such as acne, eczema, or psoriasis. Keep a food journal: write down everything you eat and how your feel 1 hour afterward for 7 days. Include meals, snacks, and drinks. Observe and jot down any fluctuations in your energy level or symptoms such as headaches, muscle pain, or nasal congestion after eating certain foods. Most important, note how your skin changes: when do you see dryness, breakouts, puffiness, or rashes? Over the course of a week, you should be able to determine if certain foods are irritants for you.

Removing problem foods from your diet can dramatically improve chronic skin conditions such as acne, eczema, or psoriasis.

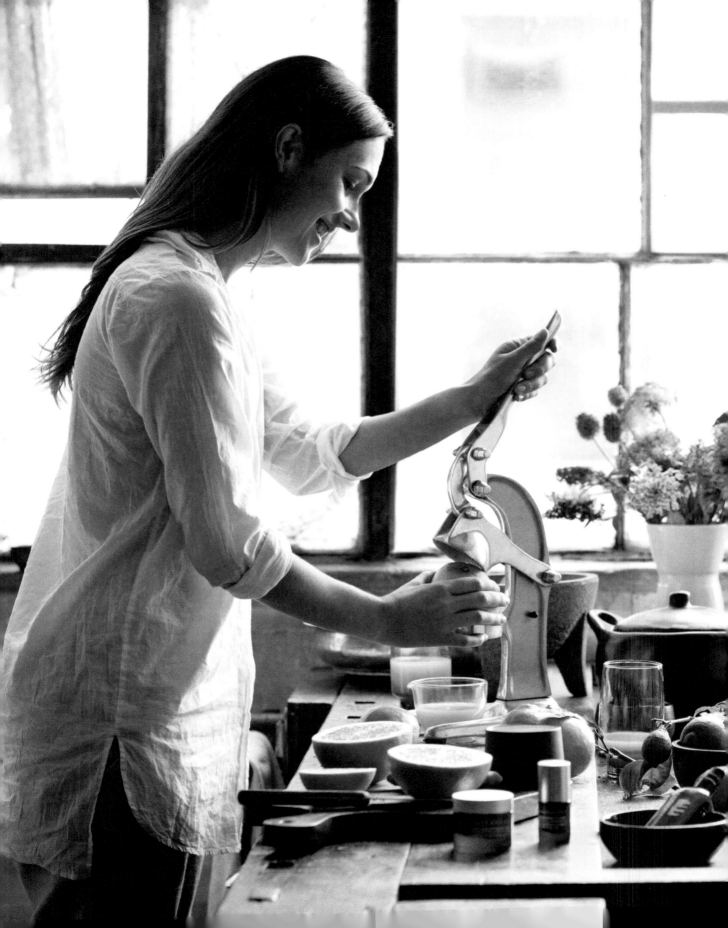

BEAUTY FOODS

Eating well for healthy skin means eating foods rich in antioxidants and essential fatty acids as well as probiotic foods, all of which will have a cleansing and anti-inflammatory effect on the body. Not surprisingly, this means eating lots of plants, just like our ancient ancestors did foraging in their natural environment.

The basic rule is to fill your plate mostly with a variety of organic fresh vegetables and legumes (beans and peas), then add a smaller amount of whole grains (brown rice, amaranth, quinoa, or barley, not refined white flour or rice). If you are not a vegetarian, include a small portion (3 to 4 ounces) of clean protein such as organic beef, free-range poultry, pastured pork, wild game, or oily fish such as wild salmon.

To really boost your skin fitness and to counteract the fact that you may have overindulged in the wrong foods, increase your intake of the foods in the following sections to protect the body from oxidative damage, keep your gut microbiome robust and prevent inflammation.

Phytonutrients

Plants are rich in antioxidants, vitamins, and minerals and when consumed, help to clean up cellular damage caused by compounds called free radicals. You can promote these benefits by zeroing in on a diet that includes 2 to 3 cups of vegetables daily. Before you freak out, this is not as difficult as it seems. Drinking a green juice daily will meet roughly a third of your requirements. Opt for a salad at lunchtime or look for soups that have lots of veggies. At dinner, include two vegetable side dishes and you are done.

Cruciferous vegetables are especially beneficial for healthy skin, since they contain sulfuric compounds called glucosinolates that are potent detoxifiers for the liver. Vegetables rich in beta-carotene such as beets, carrots, or sweet potatoes are loaded with antioxidants; note, these need to be consumed in moderation as they are also high in sugar.

Fruit is high in antioxidants but is also high in sugar, which can spike inflammation, so go easy. Avocados are excellent for the skin and contain a lot of the good fats discussed below. Try to eat as many raw foods as you can, as these vegetables and fruits naturally have enzymes that are detoxifying for the body and tame inflammation.

Herbs and spices are also a good source of phytonutrients. Cilantro is rich in vitamin A, while parsley is loaded with vitamin C. Garlic has strong antimicrobial properties that help to keep the gut flora in balance. Rosemary and turmeric are both rich in antioxidants and are also anti-inflammatory. Add 1 teaspoon of fresh herbs and spices to your dishes to boost flavor as well as health benefits, and explore incorporating additional skin-friendly herbs (see pages 136–137).

Fiber

Consuming empty foods that lack fiber or roughage leads to constipation. In turn, constipation encourages toxicity, since it increases the length of time food stays in the intestines.

Eating dietary fiber helps reduce the amount of time potentially damaging substances are in contact with the intestinal surfaces—especially heavy metals from the environment that are processed by the liver—by encouraging increased bowl motion. Another benefit of fiber is that it feeds billions of bacteria in our gut (see below).

The skin, along with the liver and kidneys, is an organ of detoxification. When the liver becomes overwhelmed with toxins, the skin will show signs of inflammation such as redness, bumps, or blemishes. By consuming 25 to 30 grams of fiber a day, which is abundant in whole grains, dark leafy greens, beans, and crunchy vegetables, both your liver and gut will work more efficiently to help keep your skin healthy.

Probiotics and Prebiotics

Probiotics are healthy bacteria that nurture the gut flora, the natural bacterial content of the intestines, by recolonizing it with organisms to defend against harmful bacteria, viruses, or yeast. Prebiotics are plant carbohydrates that nourish the good bacteria in the intestines by helping them grow, improving the good-to-bad bacteria ratio. The endothelial lining of the intestines is semipermeable and can easily be compromised by poor food choices, heavy use of over-the-counter pain medications, and stress. Probiotics are key to good skin since they protect the gut lining, boost nutrient assimilation, and thereby prevent inflammation. Recent studies even suggest that a healthy gut not only promotes improved overall immunity but also mediates a number of stress-related conditions including anxiety and depression.

While it may seem easier to take a probiotic supplement to help nurture the gut microflora, fermented foods (see chart, page 101), rich in enzymes and friendly bacteria, are a better choice and are easy to incorporate in your diet. Nature provides vital energies in foods that are a superior choice, while supplementation with probiotics can be difficult to ensure potency. Save probiotic supplements for travel, stressful times, or other times when finding fermented foods is difficult.

Good Fats

In our phobia over fat, we often neglect the fact that there are some beneficial fats our body, and especially our skin, needs in order to be healthy. The bad ones are hydrogenated fats, which are found in a lot of mainstream processed foods like crackers and snack foods.

Essential fatty acids (EFAs) are a type of fatty acid found in many good oils that cannot be produced in the body and must be obtained through diet or supplementation. EFAs come in two forms: omega-3s and omega-6s. The omega-3s primarily contain alpha-linolenic acid and the omega-6s contain linoleic acid and gamma-linolenic acid. Linoleic acid helps skin cells maintain water as well as build dermal ceramides, which are the binding agents between skin cells that give them firmness and tonicity. Gamma-linolenic acid (GLA) is critical in supporting healthy cell membranes and maintaining barrier function by keeping moisture locked in and toxins locked out.

Omega-3 and omega-6 essential fatty acids must be consumed in the right amounts to have a healthy body. Modern diets are rich in omega-6s, which are found in refined vegetal oils used in fast or processed foods and are pro-inflammatory. Research estimates that most people consume over ten times the amount of omega-6 over omega-3 foods that they should.

In contrast, omega-3 fats come primarily from cold-water fish and reduce inflammation. The best source of omega-3s are oily fish such as sardines, mackerel, and salmon (make sure that you eat wild salmon and not farm raised, which are not only loaded with antibiotics in order to endure captivity but also have high levels of PCBs, a carcinogenic chemical, due to the feed they ingest). Other sources of omega-3s include grass-fed meat and free-range eggs. In the plant kingdom, flaxseed, evening primrose, black currant, and borage seed oil all contain omega-3s (these last three oils are beneficial to the skin topically as well). Omega-3s are especially helpful for strengthening the skin barrier to resist inflammation, making them an important ally in treating aggravated skin conditions such as eczema, psoriasis, or acne.

Probiotics are key to good skin since they protect the gut lining, boost nutrient assimilation, and thereby prevent inflammation.

**Moderately
Alkaline Foods**
Almond Milk
Brussel Sprouts
Cauliflower
Coconut
Grapefruit
Quinoa
Squash
Tofu

Highly Alkaline
Avocado
Broccoli
Cucumber
Garlic
Green Drinks
Kale
Parsley
Spinach
Tomato

Moderately Acidic
Apple
Banana
Berries
Goat Cheese
Grapes
Rice (Brown, Wild)
Ocean Fish
Walnuts

Highly Acidic
Alcohol
Beef
Cheese
Chicken
Coffee
Eggs
Farmed Fish
Milk
Rice (White)

Skin Food

Another essential skin food that helps to combat inflammation is Flax-seed. Flaxseed is an excellent source of EFAs and should be added to you diet as often as possible. In order to reap the benefits of flaxseed oil, keep the bottle refrigerated and add a teaspoon to salad dressings.

Another smart way to get a boost of EFAs is to stock a peppermill with whole flaxseeds and grind them as needed into soups, salads, or your favorite entrée. Keep the peppermill in the fridge to keep the flaxseeds fresh.

If time is an issue, you can take an herbal supplement to balance your diet. Take black currant oil in doses of 500 milligrams two times a day.

ALKALINE FOODS

Diets rich in acid or acid-forming foods such as meat, cheese, processed foods, alcohol, and coffee promote inflammation in the body over time. Signs of acidity include chronic fatigue, muscle and joint stiffness, allergies, and sensitized skin. Not surprisingly, sleep deprivation, lack of exercise, and stress accelerate acidity. To give your skin the glow that it craves, eat more alkaline foods—primarily the plant-based foods we have already discussed—as well as alkaline-forming foods such as lemon. Although lemon is naturally acidic, once it enters the body, it becomes alkalizing and is the perfect way to balance someone who is in an acidic state. A key element of the Naturopathica holistic skin care regimen is to drink a glass of lemon water each morning to alkalize the body as well as to stimulate the colon and liver to release waste. Fermented foods such as sauerkraut and coconut yogurt are another excellent source of alkalinity. Try to make your diet 60 to 75 percent alkaline foods if you are prone to sensitive or blemished skin.

BEAUTY FOODS

Research shows that diet influences your complexion. What you eat can affect your hormone balance, acne or inflammation, a key driver of premature aging. Nourish yourself with the foods below to look and feel your best.

NAME & ORIGIN	BEST FOOD SOURCE	INTERNAL BENEFIT	BEAUTY TIP
Alkaline Foods	Eat more raw vegetables (cooking depletes alkilizing minerals), grapefruit, lemon, black beans, lima beans, tomatoes	Calms inflammation that can lead to sensitive skin and protects bone density.	Drink a green drink (chard, cucumber, kale, parsley) daily and supplement with coconut or alkaline water.
Fiber	Artichoke, avocado, black beans, broccoli, Brussels sprouts, chia seeds, flaxseed, lentils, oatmeal, prunes	Moves food through colon and assists in liver detoxification.	Take 2 psyllium husk capsules before bed along with two 8-ounce glasses of water to gently cleanse the colon.
Good Fats *(EFAs)*	Coconut meat and oil, oily fish (wild salmon, mackeral, sardines), olive oil, chia, hemp, and flaxseeds	Boost up omega-3s to strenthen skin barrier and calm inflammation.	Eat a dozen almond or walnuts or 1 tablespoon nut butter daily.
Liquid Replenishment	Look for alkalizing liquids like green juice, tomato juice, coconut water, and kombucha	Skin cells need water to function properly. Water plumps up the skin.	Try herbal teas, which have additional health benefits, or green teas like matcha, rich in chlorophyll and a potent detoxifier.
Phytonutrients	Arugula, asparagus, avocado, berries, broccoli, Brussels sprouts, carrots, cauliflower, celery, chard, cilantro, garlic, grapefruit, kale, parsley, spinach, squash, tomato, tumeric, turnips	High antioxidant, vitamin, and mineral content. Plant foods are prebiotics; they provide food for good bacteria in the gut to thrive.	Drink a green juice daily. Eat raw foods daily—nibble on carrots throughout the day or dip in hummus. Add 1 teaspoon of fresh herbs and/or ½ teaspoon dried spices or herbs to foods.
Probiotics	Fermented foods such as coconut yogurt, kimchi, pickled vegetables (carrots, cauliflower, cucumbers), sauerkraut, miso, tempeh, and tofu	Colonize the gut with healthy bacteria to improve digestion and create glowing skin.	Drink a glass of kombucha or kefir (drinkable yogurt) daily.

SKIN FOOD SHOPPING LIST

The first step to getting yourself on the path to eating well and nourishing your skin is to fill your kitchen with healthful food options. Begin by cleaning out your cupboards and refrigerator, throwing away any processed, nutrient-poor foods that may tempt you. Most importantly, throw away all fat-free foods and convenience foods. The foods below are all low on the glycemic index. Make copies of the shopping list and use it as a template each time you go to the grocery store.

Whole Grains

- ☐ Amaranth
- ☐ Barley
- ☐ Brown or red rice
- ☐ Oatmeal
- ☐ Quinoa

Vegetables

- ☐ Arugula
- ☐ Asparagus
- ☐ Bell Peppers (all colors)
- ☐ Broccoli
- ☐ Broccoli rabe
- ☐ Brussels sprouts
- ☐ Cabbage
- ☐ Cauliflower
- ☐ Cucumber
- ☐ Leafy greens (kale, Swiss chard)
- ☐ Leeks
- ☐ Legumes (beans, peas, lentils, chickpeas)
- ☐ Lentils
- ☐ Mushrooms
- ☐ Onions, Garlic
- ☐ Spinach
- ☐ Organic soy (tofu, tempeh)

Clean Animal Protein

- ☐ Anchovies
- ☐ Sardines
- ☐ Organic grass-fed beef
- ☐ Organic free-range chicken
- ☐ Organic free-range turkey
- ☐ Pastured pork
- ☐ Watercress
- ☐ Wild salmon

Fruit

- ☐ Avocado
- ☐ Berries (blueberries, strawberries, raspberries)
- ☐ Grapefruit
- ☐ Lemons, limes
- ☐ Melons (cantaloupe, watermelon, honeydew)
- ☐ Oranges
- ☐ Papaya
- ☐ Tomatoes

Good Fats

- ☐ Almonds, almond butter
- ☐ Chia seeds
- ☐ Coconut, coconut oil
- ☐ Flaxseed
- ☐ Olives, olive oil
- ☐ Pine nuts
- ☐ Pistachios
- ☐ Pumpkin
- ☐ Sunflower seeds
- ☐ Walnuts

Herbs, Spices & Accents

- ☐ Apple cider vinegar
- ☐ Black pepper
- ☐ Cayenne
- ☐ Cilantro
- ☐ Cinnamon
- ☐ Cumin
- ☐ Garlic
- ☐ Ginger
- ☐ Parsley
- ☐ Rosemary
- ☐ Stevia
- ☐ Thyme
- ☐ Turmeric

Liquids

- ☐ Almond milk
- ☐ Coconut water or milk
- ☐ Kombucha
- ☐ Matcha

LIQUID REPLENISHMENT

Your skin is over 60 percent water. Skin cells require water to work effectively; when the skin is adequately hydrated, it is plump, elastic, and less prone to cracks that can cause inflammation. Endeavor to drink at least six to ten 8-ounce serving of liquid a day—ideally, filtered water with lemon or some of the alkaline liquids listed in the Beauty Foods chart on page 101. Many mineral waters are alkaline and also rich in minerals like magnesium and calcium, which are important for healthy skin. Herbal teas are also alkaline and have a host of therapeutic properties, depending on the herbs used.

The thing about drinking enough liquids throughout the day is that there has to be a certain amount of vigilance involved. One of the questions I ask when I take a lifestyle history from a client at our spa is, "Do you drink enough water?" Almost invariably, the response is, "Not as much as I should." When I explain the benefits provided to the body by drinking plenty of liquid nourishment, I am often amused that many times the reason given for not drinking enough is the same: "But then I will have to pee!"

Exactly. Unless you drive a FedEx truck for a living, I have little sympathy here. Think of your kidneys as giant blood purifiers, filtering out all of the toxins and inflammatory agents that are bad for you. The more you drink, the cleaner the engine, so to speak. When the urine is a light pale yellow, this signifies you are ingesting enough water. When the urine is dark and cloudy, it's time to head to the water cooler.

Now comes the thornier issue of how to make sure you drink enough water. I find the best way is to consecrate a drinking vessel. That way you know exactly how many times you have refilled it and how much water you have consumed. My choice is a simple Mason jar, for two reasons. First, there is some evidence that plastic drinking bottles have the potential to leach chemicals into the water they hold, especially when subjected to sunlight or hot water. Second, a Mason jar has a measurement system written on the glass and you can see clearly how many ounces or milliliters you consume. Also, I find that a glass vessel does not impart a plastic taste and actually keeps the water cooler.

By all means, do not limit your liquid nourishment to water. The recipes on pages 113–123 are filled with nutritive value for the skin and will keep the purification system that the kidneys provide in top form.

Supplement your 14-day Detox Plan (page 107) with the following:

Nutritional Medicine Enjoy a Moringa Matcha Latte (page 144), rich in chlorophyll, a potent detoxifier; or a Golden Turmeric Latte (page 145) blended with anti-inflammatory turmeric to help nourish a healthy gut.

Herbal Medicine Add 40 drops of milk thistle tincture (see page 147), a powerful liver-cleansing herb, to juice or green tea and drink twice a day to support proper digestive functioning. If weight loss is part of your detox goal, add 40 drops of green coffee tincture to juice or tea and drink twice daily. Green-coffee extract has been reported to assist weight loss due to chlorogenic acid, a compound that may inhibit the body's absorption of fat and glucose. To cleanse the colon from buildup of toxic material, take 1 teaspoon of psyllium husks (see page 98) before bedtime and drink two 8-ounce glasses of water for proper assimilation.

Mind-Body Detox Now is a good time to do a mental detox. Do a media fast and don't read or watch the news. Unhook from your smart phone after 6 p.m. and on the weekends. Get rid of all processed foods and create a new recipe folder of healthy meal ideas. Consult the sleep tips on page 127 to ensure a good night's rest. And don't forget meditation to clear the mind of toxic stress. Incorporate the Grounding Breath exercise (page 133) into your daily routine.

Detox

Is it possible to love eating and yet still look and feel beautiful? I believe that the answer is yes. The dilemma I face when I flip through most health and well-being books is that these authors focus too heavily on the health-promoting benefits of their regimens and seem to forget about the sheer pleasure of food. Who wants to live that way? There's too much to enjoy.

So, go ahead and enjoy yourself, indulge when you feel like it, and when things get out of balance, rely on a detox program to get you on track with the right foods again. That way, when the inevitable retox comes—when we fill up on all the wrong things—you won't panic, you'll know what to do.

Remember, the skin is one of the largest organs of detoxification. Increasing numbers of people suffer from eczema, psoriasis, and skin infections that are an inflammatory response to the buildup of toxins in the body. By cleansing the body of some of these inflammatory irritants, the clarity, texture, and appearance of your skin can improve dramatically.

If you're not sure where to start, or want some guidance as you begin your detox, use the following 14-day plan.

DETOX QUESTIONNAIRE

Detoxing brings about a healthy body, glowing skin, and a clear mind. The body can provide a host of symptoms that reflect an imbalance, from digestive disturbances and headaches to more subtle symptoms such as puffiness underneath the eyes and bad breath. Complete the following questionnaire to determine your need for detoxification. Rate the frequency with which you experience these symptoms by filling in the appropriate number for each.

Frequently   3
Moderately   2
Mildly   1
Never   0

Fatigue, fluctuations in energy even after a good night's rest _____

Headaches or migraines _____

Stiff joints, muscle pains _____

Irritability, mood swings _____

Insomnia, including inability to fall asleep or to stay asleep _____

Lowered immunity, frequent colds or flus _____

Sinus congestion or sensitivity to allergies, asthma _____

Inefficient digestion (gas, constipation, loose stools) _____

Overeating or compulsive eating _____

Low tolerance to caffeine or alcohol _____

Bloating after meals _____

Prolonged use of antibiotics _____

Skin imbalances including acne, eczema, and psoriasis _____

Dry skin, dull, flaky skin _____

Thin, ridged or split nails _____

Dark circles underneath eyes, puffiness under eyes _____

Coating on tongue, body odor, excess mucus, bad breath _____

Smoking _____

Exposure to hazardous chemicals, chemotherapy or radiation _____

Excessive drinking, drugs, or over-the-counter medicines _____

Total _____

YOUR SCORE

0–5   High Vitality
5–15   Good Vitality
15–30   Average Vitality
30–50   Low Vitality
50–70   High Burnout and Toxicity

If you are experiencing any of the above symptoms frequently or demonstrate average or low vitality, you will benefit from a detox program. Keep your score so that you can redo the questionnaire after you have completed your detox program and rate your progress.

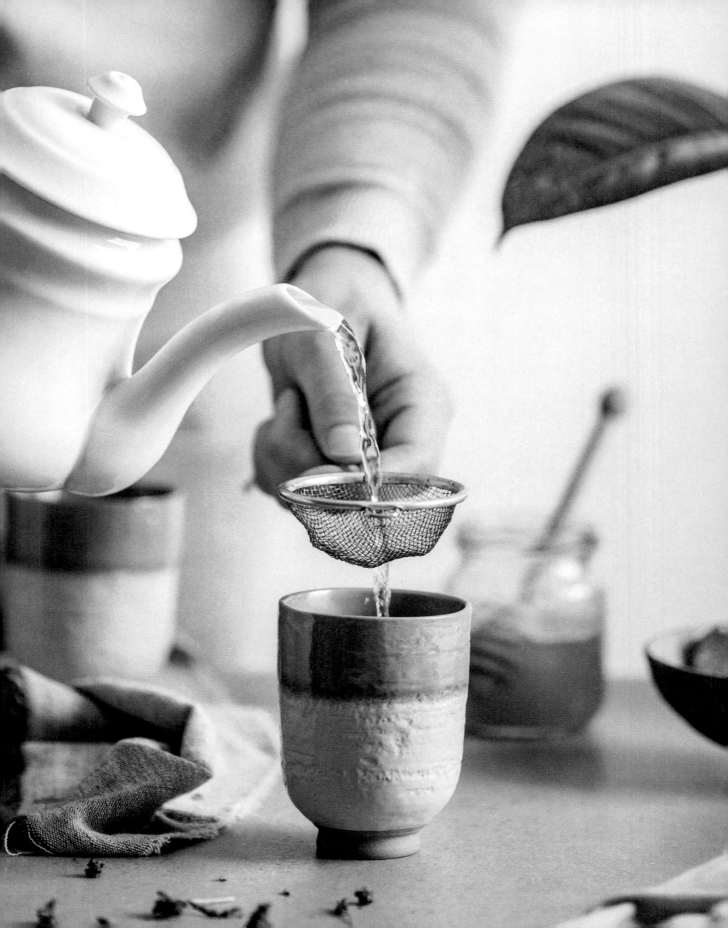

14-DAY DETOX PLAN

The main goal of a detox program is to encourage the removal of toxins already in your system and to reduce the level of new toxins you take in. The following nutritional medicine program introduces gentle, cleansing foods to increase the removal of toxins and then uses phytonutrient-rich foods to repair weak organs and tissues. This process is supported with herbal remedies and detox rituals for enhanced results.

Week 1: Rest and Cleanse

Avoid the following acidic foods: processed foods, fried foods, processed meats, sugar, alcohol, coffee, tea, soft drinks, and dairy products. Substitute the following mostly alkaline foods: steamed vegetables (especially dark leafy vegetables like Swiss chard, kale, mustard greens, and spinach) as well as fermented green veggies, which aid digestion and provide a dose of probiotics to rebalance the gut flora (see the recipe on page 101). Add fiber-rich whole-grain foods (unprocessed brown rice, quinoa, or amaranth) and clean protein derived from tofu, tempeh, eggs, or oily fish such as salmon or sardines, rich in amino acids. Snack on nuts such as almonds, walnuts, and cashews and low-sugar, enzyme-rich fruits such as papaya, grapefruit, or berries (raspberries, strawberries, blackberries).

Week 2: Repair and Renew

Continue as above, just adding more fruits and vegetables to counteract the effects of high-acid foods such as red meat and processed foods. Add free-range organic chicken, turkey, or pastured pork and more phytonutrient foods such as asparagus, leeks, sea vegetables, sprouts, squash, and zucchini. Include good fats such as avocados and olives.

Most naturopathic doctors and herbalists believe that toxins are usually stored in the fatty tissue of the body as well as in the joints. It is not uncommon during the course a detox program to feel worse for several days as these toxins are released into the system. Headaches, neck or back pains, or joint stiffness are some of the common symptoms. Do not be tempted to reach for sugar, coffee, or junk food and do increase the activation of your liver enzymes to remove the toxins by eating more cruciferous vegetables, which contain the building blocks for your liver to make glutathione, an essential antioxidant.

DETOX TIPS

- In addition to your morning lemon juice to alkalinize the system, be sure to add a daily green juice, full of antioxidants and phytochemicals to aid in cleansing your system.

- Try to cut back on cooking and eat mainly raw foods. Raw foods contain more nutrients and enzymes.

- Eat your largest meal at the middle of the day to allow proper assimilation.

- Eat consciously and slowly: do not eat while watching TV or on the run.

- Drink 2 to 3 liters per day of liquids to flush toxins out of the system, such as herbal tea—or just small amounts of kombucha or coconut water, since they contain sugar.

- Fast daily for at least 12 hours (7 p.m. to 7 a.m.).

SKIN BRUSHING

Skin brushing encourages the removal of dead skin cells, as well as stimulating circulation. This in turn increases the removal of toxins such as the by-products of cellular metabolism. Purchase a soft vegetable bristle brush, available at most health-food stores, and rub a drop of a mild essential oil like lavender (*Lavandula vera*) on the brush to sterilize it. Using a light, sweeping stroke, begin at the feet and work up the leg, front and back toward the torso. To encourage the movement of lymph flow toward the main lymphatic ducts underneath the collarbones, always stroke toward the center of the body. Brush up both sides of the arms and across the shoulders, and continue up the back and neck. Finish the treatment with small circular strokes on the abdomen in a clockwise direction, following the movement of the colon.

The following ritual is one of our most popular home bath treatments recommended at Naturopathica after our Signature Blue Eucalyptus Energizing massage. Juniper has long been known for its cleansing properties, mainly as a diuretic. Cypress is decongesting for veins and lymphatic vessels, and lemon helps to alkalize the body as well as stimulate digestion.

Detoxifying Bath and Body Oil

MAKES	4 ounces
PREP TIME	10 minutes
YOU WILL NEED	one 4-ounce dark-colored glass bottle

A	HR	SR	M

TIMESAVER TIP
Try the **Naturopathica Deep Forest Bath & Body Oil,** which uses a blend of these along with other soothing essential oils.

This ritual is one of our most popular home treatments. Fill your bathtub with hot (100°–110°F) water. Add 1 capful of the Detoxifying Bath and Body Oil to still water and disperse with your hands. Soak in the hot water for a short duration until light perspiration appears, 8 minutes maximum. Wrap yourself in a robe or towel and rest for 5 minutes to let blood pressure normalize and drink a cool, refreshing glass of mineral water with lemon.

4 ounces carrier oil (select one of the carrier oils on pages 60–61)

10 drops juniper (*Juniperus communis*) essential oil

18 drops lemon (*Citrus limon*) essential oil

10 drops balsam fir (*Abies balsamea*) essential oil

12 drops bergamot (*Citrus aurantium bergamia*) essential oil

3 drops cypress (*Cupressus sempervirens*) essential oil

Pour half of the carrier oil into the bottle. Add the essential oils, cover tightly, and roll between you palms to disperse the oils. Open, top off with the remaining carrier oil, cover tightly again, and agitate a second time. Let sit for 1 hour.

NOTE For added detox benefits, use a body brush for lymphatic brushing before bathing (see above).

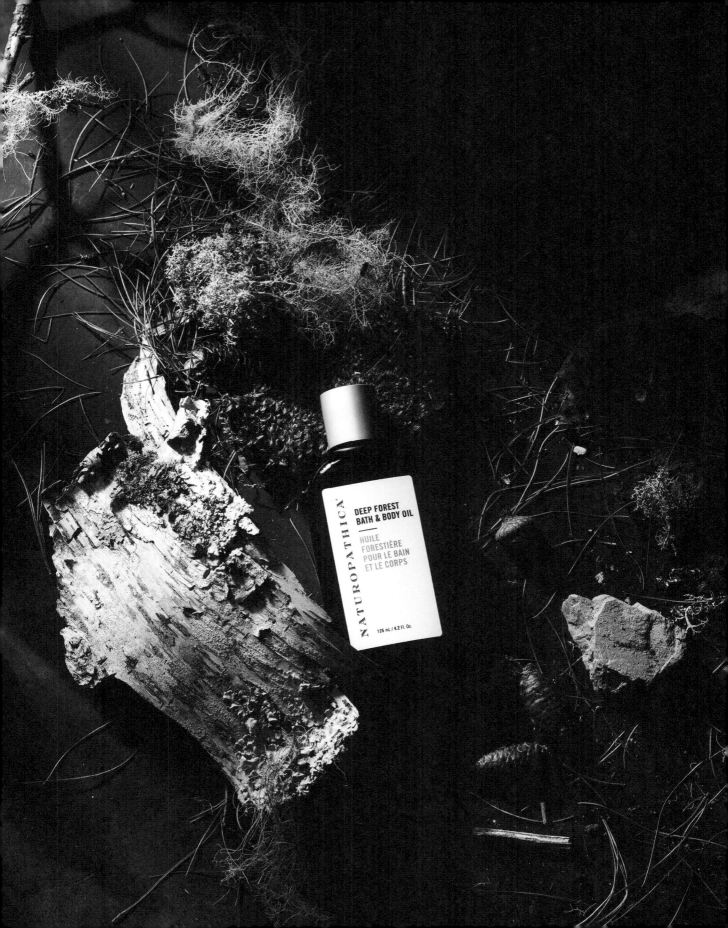

DETOX MASSAGE

Some of the most common symptoms experienced leading up to and during a detox program are poor digestion and assimilation of food. These imbalances can manifest through such symptoms as constipation, diarrhea, or bloating after meals.

Aromatherapy massage can be an effective tool in helping to calm gastric distress. Visceral massage helps tonify the abdominal organs by bringing fresh blood and nutrients, and by helping to facilitate the removal of waste material. The essential oils in the blends below have either a stimulating or antispasmodic action, depending upon the desired result.

Calming Belly Massage Oil

MAKES	1 ounce
PREP TIME	10 minutes
YOU WILL NEED	one 1-ounce glass bottle

A	HR	SR	M

TIMESAVER TIP
Try the **Naturopathica Re-Boot Aromatic Alchemy,** which uses these as well as other soothing essential oils in a jojoba carrier oil and can be applied directly on the body.

This calming oil and massage provides relief from abdominal bloating, rumbling, or diarrhea.

1 ounce carrier massage oil (select one of the carrier oils on pages 60–61)

7 drops peppermint (Mentha piperita) essential oil

3 drops lemongrass (Santalum album) essential oil

2 drops holy basil (Ocimum sanctum) essential oil

Pour half of the carrier oil into the bottle. Add the essential oils, cover the bottle tightly, and roll between your palms to disperse the oils. Open, top off with the remaining carrier oil, cover tightly again, and agitate a second time. Let sit for 1 hour.

Pour a small amount of the massage oil into your hands and rub your hands together to warm the oil. Place your palms underneath your nose and take 3 deep inhalation breaths to allow the essential oils to assimilate into the bloodstream via the respiratory tract.

Begin by massaging the belly in a counterclockwise direction. Using the pads of your fingers, sink into the soft tissue just below the right lower rib. Make small circular movements with your fingertips and continue downwards along the perimeter of the belly, first downwards, then moving across the lower abdomen just above the groin, proceeding up along the opposite ribcage and finally across the top of the abdomen, then down until you reach the starting place. Repeat this same movement, making smaller circles as you continue, until you reach your belly button.

Finish the treatment with a relaxing warm compress that will increase the absorption of the essential oils. Soak a hand towel in hot water and apply over the belly. Breathe deeply and relax while the essential oils penetrate.

Stimulating Belly Massage Oil

This stimulating oil and massage provides relief from constipation.

1 ounce carrier massage oil (select one of the carrier oils on pages 60–61)

5 drops sweet orange *(Citrus aurantium)* **essential oil**

4 drops cardamom *(Elettaria cardamomum)* **essential oil**

3 drops sandalwood *(Santalum album)* **essential oil**

MAKES	1 ounce
PREP TIME	10 minutes
YOU WILL NEED	one 1-ounce glass bottle

A   HR   SR   M

TIMESAVER TIP
Try the **Naturopathica Meditation Aromatic Alchemy,** which uses these as well as other stimulating essential oils in a jojoba carrier oil and can be applied directly on the body.

Pour half of the carrier oil into the bottle. Add the essential oils, cover the bottle tightly, and roll it between your palms to disperse the oils. Open, top off with remaining carrier oil, cover tightly again, and agitate a second time. Let sit for 1 hour.

Pour a small amount of oil into your hands and rub your hands together to warm the oil. Place your palms underneath your nose and take 3 deep inhalation breaths to allow the essential oils to assimilate into the bloodstream via the respiratory tract.

Begin by massaging the belly in a clockwise direction. Using the pads of your fingers, sink into the soft tissue just below the right lower rib. Make small circular movements with your fingertips and continue upwards along the ribcage and then down the opposite ribcage until just above the groin. Continue across the belly and then up the opposite side until you reach the starting place. Repeat this same movement, making smaller circles as you continue, until you reach your belly button.

Finish the treatment with a relaxing warm compress that will increase the absorption of the essential oils. Soak a hand towel in hot water and apply over the belly. Breathe deeply and relax while the essential oils penetrate.

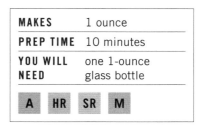

HEALING FOODS

Use the recipes that follow as an essential part of any detox plan to restore your mind and body. These foods will help mitigate the effects of your latest binge without depriving you of the pleasure of eating delicious food.

Detox Soup

Miso, a flavorful paste made from fermented soybeans and grains, has myriad health benefits. There are several varieties—soybean, rice, or barley—any of which can be used for this recipe. Traditionally served in Japan as a tonic for stomach or liver ailments, miso is a useful probiotic to rebalance the gut flora.

MAKES	1 serving
PREP TIME	20 minutes

A	HR	SR	M

1 tablespoon miso paste

1 cup boiling water

½ cup soft tofu, cut into small pieces

2 scallions, thinly sliced

Optional additions: Add watercress leaves as a cleanser for the liver. For a heartier soup, add soba, a gluten-free Japanese noodle available at health-food stores.

Place the miso in a heatproof bowl. Add ¼ cup of the boiling water and stir to make a paste. Stir in the remaining water as well as all the remaining ingredients you are using. Serve hot.

Dandelion Detox

Dandelion is one of the most important liver cleansing herbs and is useful in skin care to clear up congestion or irritation found in Hormone Reactive or Stress Reactive skin (see pages 36 and 40). Dandelion is high in vitamins A and C as well as rich in minerals such as magnesium. This recipe may seem a strange combination, but trust me, it is as delicious as it is nutritious. Tomatoes and watermelon are good sources of lycopene, a carotenoid antioxidant that is good for the skin and alkalinizing for the body. Dandelions are bitter herbs but here, the watermelon helps mask the flavor.

MAKES	1 serving
PREP TIME	30 minutes

A	HR	SR	M

½ cup dandelion greens

2 pounds watermelon, rinds removed, cut into chunks

¾ cup chopped fresh tomatoes

1 tablespoon fresh lemon juice

Feed the dandelion greens, watermelon, and tomatoes into a juicer. Stir in the lemon juice and serve.

Tropical Green Smoothie

MAKES	2 servings
PREP TIME	10 minutes

A	HR	SR	M

Although green smoothie drinks are lauded by the beauty press, I am suspicious of these beverages. While I understand the benefits of adding leafy greens to drinks to enhance health benefits, oftentimes the results taste like you did a face plant onto your lawn. Call me crazy, but wheatgrass juice makes me gag.

Then I went to visit one of our spa partners, the Lodge at Woodloch, and was fortunate enough to be invited to a Beauty Foods lecture hosted by the holistic nutritionist Talia Segal Fidler. Talia is a master at combining good nutrition with great taste. This green smoothie drink is proof in practice, and packs more nutrients into one drink than can be consumed in a single-serving salad. Avocado is rich in omega-3 fatty acids and antioxidants, and the greens help to detoxify. For an extra kick to start your day, add the **Naturopathica Stress Resistance Honey,** fortified with adaptogenic herbs such as Siberian ginseng and schisandra berry.

½ avocado

1 cup fresh or frozen chopped mango

2 handfuls of dark leafy greens such as Swiss chard, kale, or spinach, stems removed

½ cucumber, sliced

Juice of 1 lime

One 1-inch piece ginger, peeled and sliced

1 or 2 Medjool dates, pitted

1 cup almond milk, preferably homemade (page 115) or unsweetened coconut water

1 tablespoon chia seeds (optional)

1 tablespoon Naturopathica Stress Resistance Honey (optional)

¼ cup ice cubes, if needed

Combine all of the ingredients in a blender and blend until smooth. Add the ice cubes if more liquid is needed. Pour into a tall glass and serve immediately.

NOTE You can substitute fresh or frozen blueberries, strawberries, banana, pineapple, etc., for the mango.

Homemade Almond Milk

Homemade almond milk is more nutritious than commercial versions. It is also sweeter, as it loses some of the honey-like notes when it is pasteurized, along with beneficial antioxidants, phenols, and flavonoids. This delicious creamy, nutty plant milk takes only minutes to make and is the perfect base for Golden Turmeric Lattes (page 145), smoothies, or matcha due to its natural alkalizing properties. If you choose, you can add coconut oil to this blend. Virgin coconut oil is rich in lauric acid, which boosts immunity and fights infection, and can be useful for Stress Reactive skin personalities that are prone to broken, cracked skin.

MAKES	3 servings
PREP TIME	20 minutes

A	HR	SR	M

3 cups water

1 cup almonds, soaked for at least 4 hours, strained, and rinsed

3 pitted Medjool dates

1 teaspoon vanilla extract

¼ teaspoon ground cinnamon

Pinch of salt

1 tablespoon extra-virgin coconut oil, melted (optional)

Place the water and almonds in a blender and blend until smooth. Pour the mixture into a bowl or measuring jar through a strainer lined with cheesecloth and squeeze out any remaining liquid by hand. Discard the solids. Rinse the blender and pour the strained milk back into the jar. Add the rest of the ingredients and blend thoroughly.

NOTE The almond milk will keep, refrigerated, for 3 to 5 days. You may also freeze in ice-cube trays and add to smoothies or herbal lattes as needed.

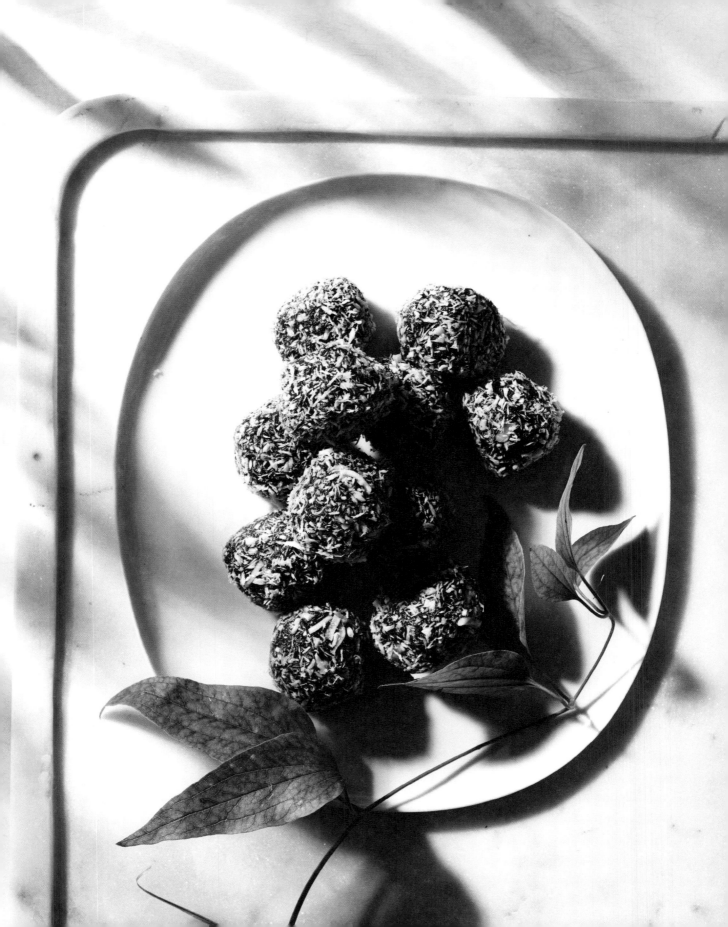

Vitality Bites

I first discovered this amazing herbal remedy when I was in school getting my master's degree in herbal medicine. A fellow student posted a recipe for energy bites to help us get through final exams. There are dozens of ways to ingest herbal remedies—teas, tinctures, or fortified honey, for example—but this herbal supplement, in my view, is the grand prize winner, because it is as delicious as it is good for you. The base of the mix is made with a nut butter, a sweetener, and a blend of tonic herbs that can be taken over a long period of time and have no side effects. This recipe uses reishi, an adaptogen herb that builds stamina and resistance to stress, along with turmeric and a dash of cayenne to reduce inflammation in the body. A dusting of matcha is added for its antioxidant benefits.

MAKES	25 bites
PREP TIME	30 minutes

A   HR   SR   M

1 cup almond butter

½ cup wildflower honey

3 tablespoons reishi powder

1 teaspoon ground turmeric

¼ teaspoon cayenne pepper

¼ teaspoon matcha powder

About 4 tablespoons carob powder

½ cup finely shredded coconut

Combine the almond butter and honey in a large bowl. Add the reishi, turmeric, cayenne, and matcha 1 tablespoon at a time, stirring constantly until evenly mixed. Sprinkle in the carob powder 1 tablespoon at a time, just until the mixture reaches a firm consistency.

Mold the mixture into balls about 1 inch in diameter by rolling pieces between your palms. Once formed, roll in the shredded coconut shreds to cover and place in a storage container lined with parchment paper. Store tightly covered in the refrigerator for up to 3 months.

Sardine Pâté

MAKES	2 servings
PREP TIME	20 minutes

A	HR	SR	M

This pâté contains sardines and anchovies—both nutritious dark, oily fish—along with walnuts, all rich in omega-3 essential fatty acids. This can be a quick and easy lunch or served as an appetizer for a main meal.

One 4-ounce can boneless sardines, packed in oil

2 anchovy fillets

1 tablespoon walnuts

1 small red onion, finely chopped

1 small clove garlic, minced

1 tablespoon capers

1 tablespoon fresh parsley

1 tablespoon white wine vinegar

1 tablespoon fresh lemon juice

Combine all of the ingredients in a food processor and purée for 15 seconds. Serve with salad greens or with rice or rye crackers. Squeeze additional lemon juice on top, if desired.

Broiled Salmon with Orange-Miso Glaze

MAKES	2 servings
PREP TIME	30 minutes

A	HR	SR	M

The omega-3 group of essential fatty acids found in oily fish such as salmon all contain potent anti-inflammatory compounds to help prevent free-radical damage. The miso and ginger both work to help nurture the intestinal micro-flora. Think of this recipe as an omega-3 booster to rejuvenate your skin.

One 3-inch piece ginger

2 tablespoons fresh orange juice

2 tablespoons mirin

3 tablespoons miso

Two 8-ounce wild salmon fillets, skinned

1 tablespoon extra-virgin olive oil

Salt

Preheat the broiler.

Peel and grate the ginger over a small bowl, squeezing the pulp with your hands to extract all the juice. Discard the pulp. Add the orange juice, mirin, and miso to the bowl. Mix well. Set aside.

Brush the top of salmon with the olive oil, sprinkle with salt, and place in a baking pan lined with aluminum foil. Place under the broiler for 2 minutes. Remove from the oven, carefully turn the fish, and continue to broil until the fish just begins to brown, about 2 minutes longer. Remove from the oven, brush the glaze on the fish, and return to the broiler for 1 minute more. Serve immediately.

Burdock Root Kimchi

A staple of Korean cuisine, this dish is traditionally made from fermented cabbage and spices. This recipe adds burdock root, which, in addition to its pleasantly crunchy texture and mildly sweet flavor, also possesses anti-inflammatory and antibacterial properties. It is a powerhouse of an antioxidant, with phenolic acids that can protect cells from free-radical damage. In Chinese medicine, burdock is considered a cooling herb and good for conditions of heat such as eczema, psoriasis, or acne. Traditionally, burdock is referred to as a blood cleanser as it strengthens the kidneys and the liver and thereby helps clarify the skin. Here burdock is paired with other antimicrobial and stimulating herbs, including garlic and ginger, to aid digestion.

MAKES	1 quart
PREP TIME	30 minutes
YOU WILL NEED	one 1-quart canning jar with lid

A HR SR M

1 pound burdock root

Zest and juice of 1 lemon

½ pound daikon radish, cut into matchsticks

Red pepper flakes to taste (optional)

1½ tablespoons unrefined sea salt or ½ cup fish sauce

¼ red bell pepper, seeded and thinly sliced

1 bunch scallions, tender green parts included, cut into 1-inch pieces

3 cloves garlic, minced

1 tablespoon peeled and finely grated fresh ginger

Peel the burdock and cut into thin slices. Place in a large bowl and squeeze the lemon juice over all to prevent oxidation and browning. Add the lemon zest, radish, and red pepper flakes to taste, if using, to the bowl and stir to combine thoroughly. Sprinkle in 1 tablespoon of the salt or $1/3$ cup of the fish sauce and mix well. Cover and let sit for 30 minutes until brine appears at the bottom of the bowl. Taste the mixture; it should have a slightly salty taste but it should not be overpowering. Add more salt or fish sauce as needed.

Fold in the bell pepper, scallions, garlic, and ginger and massage the mixture for a few minutes until everything is well combined and the brine collects again at the bottom of the bowl. Place the vegetables in the canning jar and use an instrument to compact the kimchi until the brine rises to cover the vegetables. Leave at least 1 inch of headspace at the top and screw the lid on tightly.

Place the jar on a plate or towel away from direct sunlight and leave to ferment at room temperature for 5 to 14 days. Check the jar daily, and, if necessary, press down on the vegetables with a clean spoon to keep them submerged under the brine and to release gasses produced during fermentation. The kimchi is ready when it is pleasingly sour, the flavors have mingled, and the pungency of the kimchi spices has developed. Store tightly closed in the refrigerator for up to 1 year.

Herbal Probiotic Sauerkraut

MAKES	1 quart
PREP TIME	60 minutes
YOU WILL NEED	one 1-quart canning jar with lid

A   HR   SR   M

The practice of lactic-acid fermentation, a process of converting simple or complex sugars into fermented foods, has a long history in many cultures. Homemade sauerkraut is extraordinarily rich in beneficial bacteria, the friendly organisms that help colonize the gut and, as a result, the immune system, and clarify the skin.

Store-bought sauerkraut is not raw; it is heated and pasteurized and has therefore lost most vitamin C content and enzymes. Lactic-acid fermentation makes the cabbage more easily digestible and increases food enzymes and vitamins. Caraway seeds are powerful antioxidants that help neutralize free radicals from the body and also aid digestion. Enjoy this herbal sauerkraut as a side dish alongside vegetables, or use as a condiment for sandwiches or roll ups.

2 pounds organic cabbage (white or red)

4 teaspoons kosher salt

2 tablespoons caraway seeds

Remove the large outer leaves from the cabbage and set aside. Cut the cabbage into quarters and remove the cores. Using a food processor or mandoline, shred the cabbage into strips about ¼ inch wide. Place the cabbage in a bowl and add the salt. Using your hands, massage and squeeze the cabbage thoroughly until there is a visible puddle of water in the bottom of the bowl (if you allow the cabbage to sit with the salt for 20 minutes before mixing, it will help to soften the cabbage). Add the caraway seeds and toss to distribute evenly.

Pack the mixture into the canning jar, using your fist or a utensil to compress the mixture and leaving about 2 inches of space at the top. Make sure all of the cabbage is submerged under the brine to prevent any spoilage. Add a top layer of the reserved whole cabbage leaves to fill the jar and ensure an airtight fit. Seal the jar tightly and place on a small plate or towel. Allow the sauerkraut to ferment at room temperature. Taste the sauerkraut every few days and refrigerate it when it is as sour as you like. This will stop the fermentation process. The finished sauerkraut will keep in the fridge for 6 months and up to 1 year.

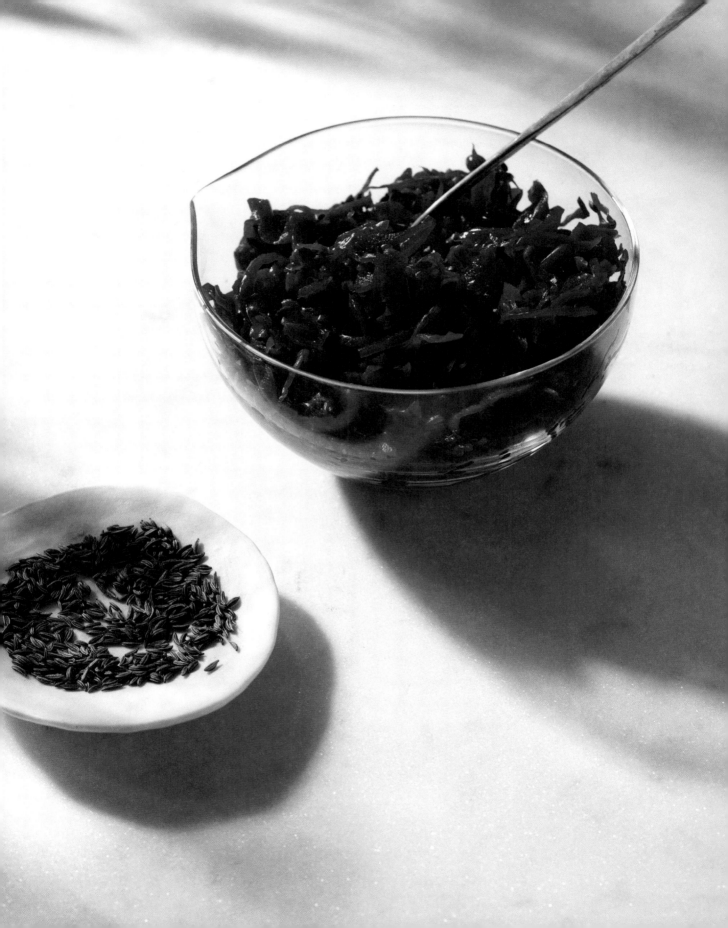

Beauty Bone Broth

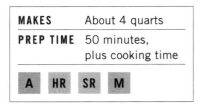

| MAKES | About 4 quarts |
| PREP TIME | 50 minutes, plus cooking time |

ADD AN ADAPTOGEN

For an extra boost, I like to add astragulus root to my Beauty Bone Broth, an adaptogen herb that grows in northern China and helps protect the body against stress, colds, and flus. Some studies suggest that astragulus helps stimulate the liver as well as lower blood sugar, possibly making it a useful ally for those with Hormone Reactive skin (see page 36).

One of the world's oldest healing foods, bone broth is rich in compounds that support healthy skin. Don't be fooled by commercial varieties of bone broth that often use bouillon cubes or powders. It is the simmering of the bones and cartilage for hours that produces a broth rich in healing compounds that promote healthy skin, hair, and nails.

The collagen in this bone broth helps heal and seal the gut lining, while minerals such as calcium magnesium and phosphorus in chicken are great for brain health. Chicken also contains the amino acids glycine, proline, and arginine, all of which have anti-inflammatory properties. Serve as the base for a soup or stew or enjoy straight up as a warm and refreshing beverage.

One 2–3-pound whole organic chicken

1 large onion, unpeeled, coarsely chopped

2 large carrots, scrubbed but unpeeled, cut into thirds

3 celery sticks, coarsely chopped

6 cloves of garlic, coarsely chopped

Several sprngs of fresh thyme, tied together

1 bay leaf

One 8-inch strip of kombu

6 black peppercorns

4 quarts cold filtered water, plus more if needed

2 strips of astragulus root (optional)

1 bunch fresh parsley and/or 1 bunch fresh dill

Sea salt

Cut the chicken into serving pieces: breasts, thighs, legs, and wings. Also keep the back bones and neck. If you can purchase chicken feet, use these as well, since they are naturally rich in collagen.

In a large stockpot, combine all of the chicken pieces, the onion, carrots, celery, garlic, thyme, bay leaf, kombu, and peppercorns. Add the water, cover, and bring to a boil, using a large spoon to remove any scum or fat that rises to the top. Reduce the heat to maintain a gentle simmer, cover, and cook for 2 hours.

Remove the chicken from the pot, and separate the meat from the bones. Set aside the meat for another dish. Place the bones back in the pot, add the astragulus root, and continue to simmer. Continue to simmer until the stock is nicely flavorful, about 6 hours longer, or up to 24 hours at a very gentle simmer. Add more water if too much liquid seems to be cooking away. The longer you cook the stock, the richer and more flavorful it will be.

A few hours before finishing the stock, add the parsley and/or dill for added flavors. Season with salt to taste. When done, remove the bones and vegetables with a slotted spoon, and strain the stock through a fine-mesh sieve. Let cool to room temperature and make sure to refrigerate within 4 hours. The next day, spoon off and discard any fat that has risen to the surface. Refrigerate for up to 3 days, or freeze in single-batch containers (ice-cube trays make nice portions for sauces, etc.) for up to 3 months.

Sea Mineral Broth

Versatile, delicious, and nutrient-dense, this mineral broth is perfect for vegetarians or anyone looking to give their body a nourishing boost. This seaweed-rich broth is fortified with a high concentration of vitamins, minerals, amino acids, and antioxidants. Sipping this stock is like giving your body an internal spa treatment. Kombu is packed with folate, magnesium, and potassium along with other trace minerals. Bladderwrack is rich in iodine as well as beta-carotene and mucilage. Reishi mushrooms have strong anti-inflammatory properties and also help protect the liver.

MAKES	6 to 7 quarts
PREP TIME	30 minutes

A HR SR M

3 large carrots, stems included, unpeeled, cut into chunks

1 leek, white and tender green parts, cut into chunks and rinsed well

2 onions, unpeeled, coarsely chopped

5 garlic cloves, unpeeled

3 dried reishi mushroom caps

1 celery root, peeled and coarsely chopped, 1 head of celery, coarsely chopped

1 garnet yam or sweet potato with skin on, scrubbed and quartered

1 bunch fresh parsley

½ bunch fresh dill

Several sprigs of fresh thyme, tied together

2 bay leaves

One 8-inch strip of kombu or Bladderwrack

8 black peppercorns

4 whole allspice berries (optional)

8 quarts cold filtered water, plus more if needed

Sea salt

Rinse all of the vegetables well, including the kombu.

In a large 12-quart stockpot, combine all of the vegetables, herbs, and spices except the sea salt. Fill the pot with water to cover the vegetables by 2 inches and bring to a boil. Reduce the heat, cover partially, and simmer for at least 2 hours and up to 4 hours. As the broth simmers, some of the liquid will evaporate. Add more water as the vegetables begin to peek out. The longer you cook the stock, the richer and more flavorful it will be.

Strain the broth through a large-mesh sieve and discard the solids. Pour the broth into heat-resistant containers and let cool at room temperature before storing. Refrigerate for up to 3 days, or freeze individual servings in containers or ice-cube trays for up to 3 months.

Chapter 5

That Which Adapts Thrives

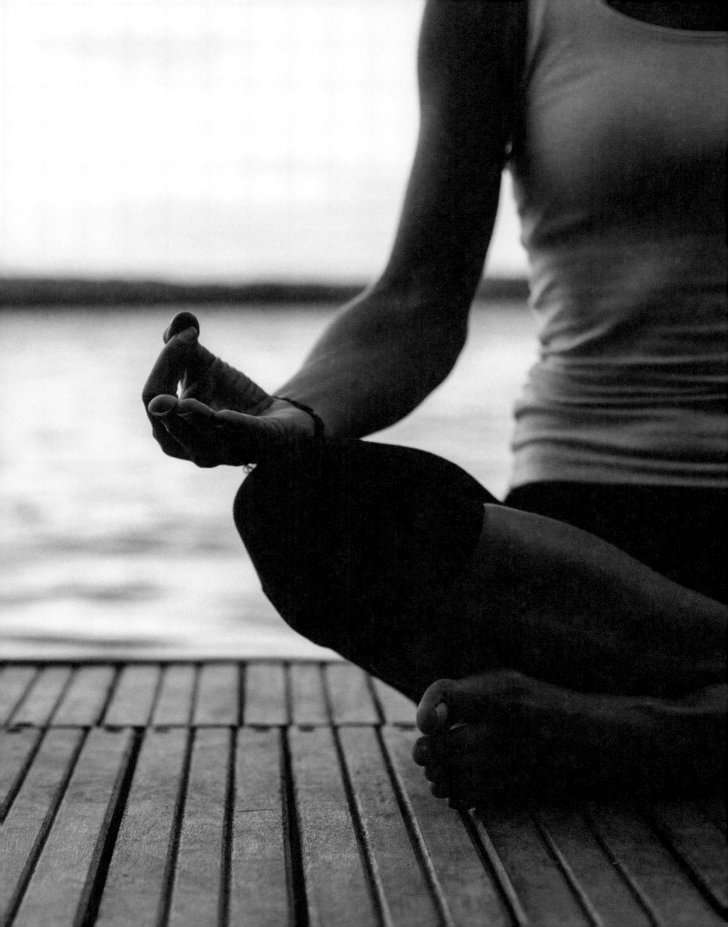

I t seems that every beauty, health, and fitness magazine you read today keeps mentioning the word "balance." To be honest, I am not really sure what they mean. To me it sounds like this nirvana-like plateau—which maybe, if I tried to really discipline myself, I could attain. Maybe if I ate more veggies or drank less wine or took a yoga class every day, then maybe I'd be in that sort of Admiral's Club for balanced people. I'm not trying to be flippant. I think there are some people who probably are quite . . . balanced. God bless them, they run Iron Man marathons, exert portion control at meals, and go to bed at a reasonable hour.

The Oxford English Dictionary defines balance as "to bring to or keep in equilibrium." The first part of that definition makes sense, but how does one maintain equilibrium? Nature, of which we are all a part, is all about cycles— ever changing, ebbing, flowing. And health is not a fixed identity, but the ability to adapt to one's environment and to the daily stress that engulfs us.

Learning to Thrive

Stress today is completely toxic. According to the National Institute of Health, 75–90 percent of all physician office visits are for stress-related complaints such as diabetes, heart disease, asthma, digestive maladies, migraines and musculoskeletal pains.[1] More alarmingly, the Center for Disease Control estimates that 11 percent of Americans take antidepressant medications, a 400 percent increase from the 1980s. For women in their 40s and 50s, the statistic is one in four.[2]

We need new ways to cope with stress. Rather than trying to prevent or balance stress, we need to learn how to adapt to it. Some stress is actually good for us. For example, research has now proven that high-intensity training is a more effective type of exercise, as short, intense workouts can increase our aerobic capacity faster and burn fat more efficiently than steady training. Severe caloric restriction is another form of beneficial stress, as studies have shown it slows the aging process and reduces the prevalence of heart disease and cancer. This phenomenon is known as the "adaptive stress response" and it is very powerful.

Herbal medicine is another way we can modulate our adaptive response to stress. Phytochemicals kick the body's cellular maintenance functions into high gear with potent antioxidants and phytochemicals like polyphenols, the bioactive compounds that upregulate our genes to keep us healthy. This allows our bodies to protect themselves from chronic inflammation and stress-related disease. The study of how our genes can be influenced by external factors is called *epigenetics* and is the future of twenty-first century wellness. This final chapter explores the idea that self-care rituals are not a form of pampering indulgence, but rather reveal how adequate sleep, herbal medicine, massage therapy, hydrotherapy, aromatherapy, and meditation can all help you to adapt to stress and rejuvenate your body.

We need new ways to cope with stress. Rather than trying to prevent or balance stress, we need to learn how to adapt to it. Some stress is actually good for us.

SLEEP

We often see visitors come to the Vitality Bar at Naturopathica Chelsea complaining of everything from fatigue, headaches, and back pain to inflamed skin and digestive problems. As part of our consultation, we ask about sleep habits. I am always amazed by how many people think good sleep is insignificant to health. Proper sleep gives your mind and body time to rest and recuperate right down to the cellular level. Medical experts say that the average American adult gets less than 6 hours sleep a night when the requirement is 8 or more. Whether your problem is falling off to sleep or not being able to sleep through the night, the following tactics will help to induce sleep.

Comfort Zone

Create an environment that is conducive to sleep. Take a tip from your ancestors and make your bedroom a cave with dark curtains or light-resistant blinds. Light exposure alters the body's internal sleep clock and effects sleep-and-wake cycles. Indulge in soft organic cotton flannel sheets in the winter or crisp organic linen sheets in summer. These luxurious natural fibers induce relaxation.

Good Sleep Habits

Develop a regular bedtime schedule. Repeating any routine night after night sends a signal to your brain that it is time to wind down. Set the stage for a good night's sleep by turning off your computer and TV as well as overhead lights an hour before bed to help you unwind. Dispense 3 or 4 drops of a calming essential oil such as lavender, neroli, or chamomile into a room diffuser or place on a tissue and slide underneath your pillowcase.

Rest and Renew

Before bed, give yourself, or exchange with a partner, a relaxing foot massage. The feet have thousands of nerve endings. Make the Tea Tree and Lemon Foot Balm (page 89) and do a foot massage featured to encourage relaxation and promote a deep sleep.

Bedtime Bath

Let the soothing properties of water be your lullaby to dreamland. Create your own relaxing bath oil using the Aromatherapy Guide on pages 66–67.

Plant Medicine

Drink a tisane, an infusion of calming and relaxing herbs and hot water, 1 hour before bedtime. Add 1 teaspoon of relaxing fresh herbs such as chamomile, lavender, and/or linden blossom. If racing thoughts are what keeps you up and anxiety is an issue, try lemon balm. For insomnia, add 40 drops of a tincture with hypnotic herbs such as passionflower, skullcap, or valerian to help promote sleep.

QUICK TIPS TO SLEEP

☐ Make lunch your biggest meal of the day, not dinner. Eat foods such as salmon or turkey that are fortified with tryptophan, an amino acid needed to promote sleep-inducing chemicals such as serotonin and melatonin.

☐ Exercise regularly. This helps control cortisol levels to help you sleep.

☐ Avoid afternoon naps longer than 20 minutes.

☐ Avoid alcohol or nicotine before bed.

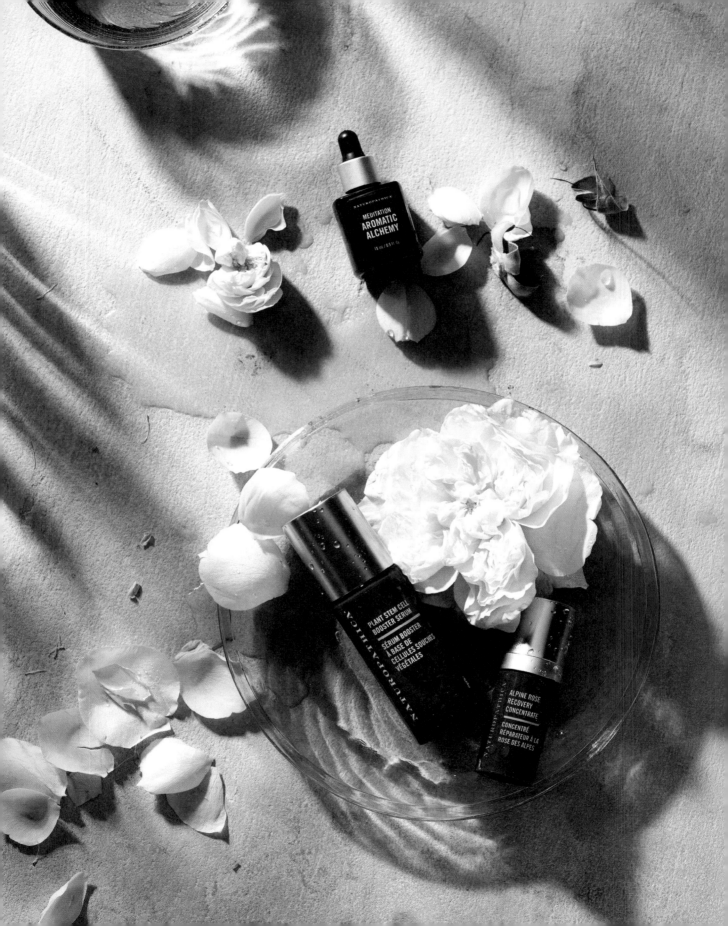

MASSAGE THERAPY

When I was growing up, my brother and sisters and I use to form a massage daisy chain in front of the TV, rubbing each other's backs. By the time the show was over, the four of us would be a column of drooling and moaning bodies pimpled with gooseflesh. The person at the front of the line would move to the back and we would begin all over again.

The renowned physician Avicenna (A.D. 980) recommended the "restorative friction" of massage for a variety of medicinal purposes. Likewise, doctors today recommend therapeutic massage for both its physical and emotional benefits. Massage improves the circulation of blood and the movement of lymph fluids, reduces blood pressure, strengthens the immune system, relieves muscle pain, and aids in relaxation of the entire body. But massage also enhances the health and nourishment of the skin. The kneading action of the flesh helps bring more oxygen and nutrients to the skin and at the same time aids in the removal of toxins. Massage is also an excellent vehicle for the absorption of therapeutic essential oils as well as the hydration of the dermis with amino acid-rich vegetal oils.

Although it may be more relaxing to receive a massage from a professional massage therapist, you can still experience the benefits of touch with a partner or through self-massage—and when you have a massage at home, you can use the very best essential oils and vegetal oils.

Following the Aromatherapy Blending Basics on pages 66–67, create a massage oil blend that best fits your mood or is designed to treat a specific condition (you will need 1 ounce for a full body massage). Then ask a partner or a friend to give and/or receive a restorative massage. When you are giving a massage, begin by having your partner lie face up on the floor or bed. Pour the oil into your hands and rub your hands together to warm the oil. Place your hands over your partner's nose and have him or her take three deep, diaphragmatic breaths in order to stimulate the relaxation response. Then gently glide, knead, and wring the muscles of affected areas throughout the body to release tension and revitalize the senses.

Just as your body benefits from a good massage, your face also benefits from enhanced circulation of blood and the movement of lymph fluids to brighten the complexion. The face has over forty muscles and regular massage helps reduce tension. Facial massage may sound like another time-consuming step in your skin care regimen, but it is actually a wonderfully relaxing nighttime beauty ritual with many benefits, even if you only practice it once or twice a week. Choose one of the facial oil recipes on pages 78–80 or follow the Aromatherapy Blending Basics on pages 66–67 to create your own serum that best suits your needs. Then try the facial protocol featured on page 81. This is the heart and soul of every holistic facial treatment at Naturopathica and is what makes our facials so popular.

PRANA EAR MASSAGE

According to traditional Chinese medicine, energy or *qi* flows through channels that can be mapped throughout the body, and each channel is paired with an organ. The pathway of the gallbladder channel wraps around the ear, and imbalances of this channel often are symptoms of toxic stress overload.

De-stress and recharge, try this self-care ritual:

Place 2 or 3 drops of bergamot essential oil into your palm, or to save time, use **Naturopathica Aromatic Alchemy.** Rub your hands briskly together, and inhale deeply to combat fatigue and ground the mind. Using the pads of your fingers on your temples, gently massage your fingers in a circular motion, moving above and around your ears to relieve tension.

Placing your thumb and index fingers behind your ears and your third finger in front, "scissor" the ears rubbing up and down for a calming effect.

Next, use your thumb and index fingers to massage the ear lobes. Continue up to the middle of the outside of the ears and gently rotate the entire ear in circles.

Complete the ritual by applying healing energy: Rub both hands briskly together until heat builds up and then cup your ears. Take several deep breaths and allow the heat to energize the senses and reinvigorate the mind.

COMPRESSES

Compresses are relaxing moist-heat treatments that are useful in increasing local circulation for dull facial complexions. You can add a compress treatment before or after a facial massage (page 81) to increase absorption of a facial serum, or try one first thing upon rising to wake up a tired mind.

Soak a washcloth in warm water, wring out, mist with a facial toner, and apply to your face. Alternatively, fill your bathroom sink with warm water. Add 2 or 3 drops of lavender, rose, or neroli essential oil and swish the water to disperse the oil. Soak the washcloth in water, wring out, and apply to your face. Inhale deeply.

BATH CURES

Hydrotherapy is an important modality of natural healing. The therapeutic use of water, including alternating hot, and cold-water treatments (baths or showers), as well as steam baths, inhalations, and compresses, all seek to strengthen the natural defenses of the body.

Warm water is sedative, promotes perspiration, and acts as an analgesic and antispasmodic for stress-induced aches and pains. Hot water draws blood to the extremities. Cold water acts as a restorative tonic to boost energy by bringing blood back to the heart. Alternating hot water with short bursts of cold water gets the blood and lymphatic fluid moving, pumping toxins out of the tissues.

Naturopathica bath cures utilize the beneficial properties of the water along with the therapeutic properties of plant extracts and essential oils. Since essential oils are lipophilic, they try to escape from water and absorb into the fatty tissue of the skin, and thus are more readily absorbed than through regular massage. Bath cures are an excellent at-home follow-up treatment to a massage or spa visit.

The therapeutic properties of the bath cure depend upon three things: the temperature of the water, the length of time the body is immersed in the water, and the types of plant extracts used. These bath cures are easy to do and will go a long way towards nourishing the principle healing systems of the body: the nervous, circulatory, lymphatic, and immune systems—all of which can affect the skin.

Detox Herbal Shower

MAKES	1 ounce
PREP TIME	10 minutes
YOU WILL NEED	one 1-ounce plastic bottle with flip lid

A	HR	SR	M

TIMESAVER TIP
Try the **Naturopathica Alpine Arnica Bath & Body Oil,** which uses these as well as a blend of other stimulating herbs.

1 ounce carrier oil (select one or a combination of the vegetal oils listed on pages 60–61)

5 drops grapefruit *(Citrus paradisi)* essential oil

4 drops rosemary *(Rosemarinus officinalis)* essential oil

3 drops bay laurel *(Laurus nobilis)* essential oil

3 drops basil *(Ocimum basilicum)* essential oil

Stand under a warm shower. After your muscles have relaxed, alternate hot and cold water (one minute hot, 15 seconds cold). Repeat three times to bring a healthy glow to skin by increasing the flow of blood and oxygen to the surface of the body. For added benefit, apply the detoxifying oil blend below to a moist washcloth to enhance circulation.

Pour half of the carrier oil into the bottle. Add the essential oils, close the bottle tightly, and roll bottle between your palms to disperse the oils. Open, top off with the remaining carrier oil. Close tightly again and agitate a second time. Let sit for at least 1 hour.

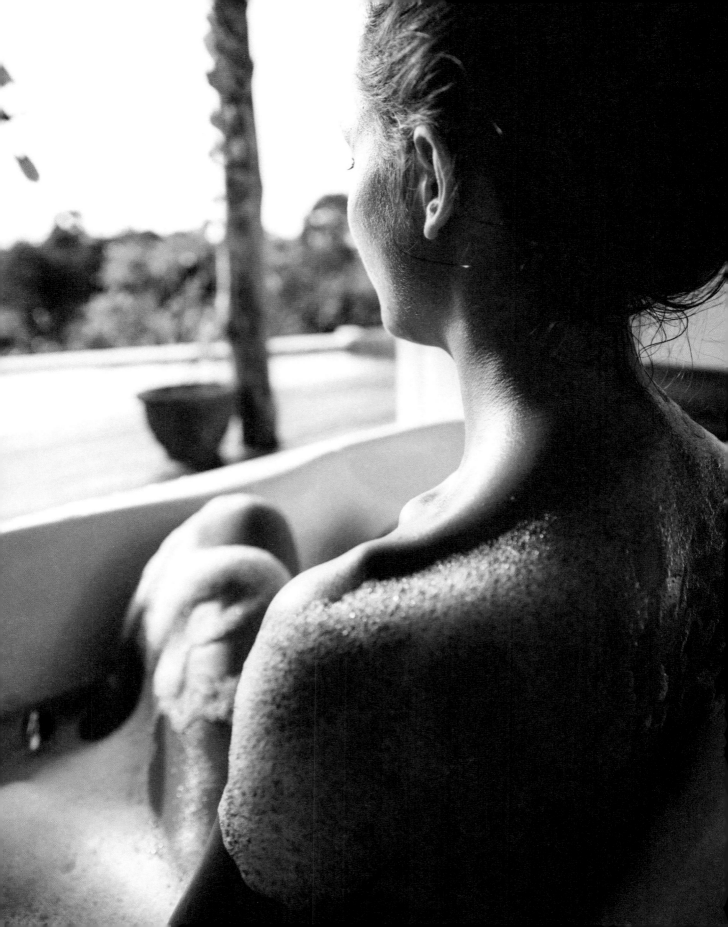

Relax Herbal Bath

MAKES	4 ounces
PREP TIME	10 minutes
YOU WILL NEED	one 4-ounce glass bottle

A **HR** **SR** **M**

This calming bath is designed to soothe daily stress-related symptoms such as nervous exhaustion, anxiety, or insomnia and is the perfect nighttime bath. Soaking in warm water relaxes the central nervous system, benefiting the body emotionally and physically.

Follow the Aromatherapy Blending Basics on pages 66–67 to create your own relaxing bath oil, or try the recipe below.

4 ounces carrier oil (select one or a combination of the vegetal oils listed on pages 42–43)

14 drops sandalwood *(Santalum album)* **essential oil**

13 drops rose *(Rosa damascena)* **essential oil**

9 drops bergamot *(Citrus aurantium Bergamia)* **essential oil**

3 drops patchouli *(Pogostemon cablin)* **essential oil**

Fill the bottle halfway with the carrier oil. Add the essential oils, close the bottle tightly, and roll it between your palms to disperse the oils. Open and top off with the remaining carrier oil. Cover tightly again and agitate a second time. Let sit for at least 1 hour.

Fill your tub with warm (92°–100°F) water. Add 1 capful of the bath oil to the water and disperse with your hands. Soak in the warm water for 20–30 minutes.

MEDITATION

There is one undeniable fact: If you want to really reduce your stress, you have to focus on the breath. This could be the reason for the growing popularity of meditation. Today more than 18 million American adults practice some form of meditation daily, twice as many as a decade ago. Let's loop back to the concept of epigenetics, that our genes can be influenced by external or environmental factors that turn genes ON or OFF. To best demonstrate how life experience can alter DNA, we need to look at telomeres, the section at each end of the chromosome that protects the chromosome from unraveling like a tip of a shoelace. As we age, our telomeres get shorter with every new division of a cell.

In the 1980s, a scientist by the name of Elizabeth Blackburn discovered an enzyme called telomerase that can protect and rebuild telomeres. Numerous research studies seem to indicate that meditation can increase the levels of telomerase anywhere from 30–40 percent.[3] For me there is no better evidence than this that biology is not our destiny. We have far greater control over our health outcomes than we have previously envisioned.

Similar to enjoying a hot shower followed by a fresh set of clothes, meditation offers us this sense of cleansing for the mind by getting rid of the clutter and putting the need to constantly be on the run on hold. This deeper level of self-awareness allows us to be more in tune with the body's needs and our true goals.

Meditating is about sitting down for some quality time with your mind, that fiendish little ferret of an organ that most times won't let you sit still for more than a nanosecond. If you find that your days are racing by you without achieving your goals, and that lately you have the attention span of a gnat, well then, meditation is your antidote.

Stress reactive skin personalities take note. Meditation not only releases neurotransmitters that shut down adrenaline, it also lowers your heart rate, boosts the immune system, and brings increased oxygen, the skin's favorite ally, into the lungs.

Twenty minutes. That's all it takes—the same amount of time you would spend applying a rejuvenating face mask. Of course, if your interests prevail, you can go on and learn more elaborate forms of meditation like Zen, Vipassana or Transcendental Meditation. But to start, try the simple Grounding Breath meditation exercise in the sidebar.

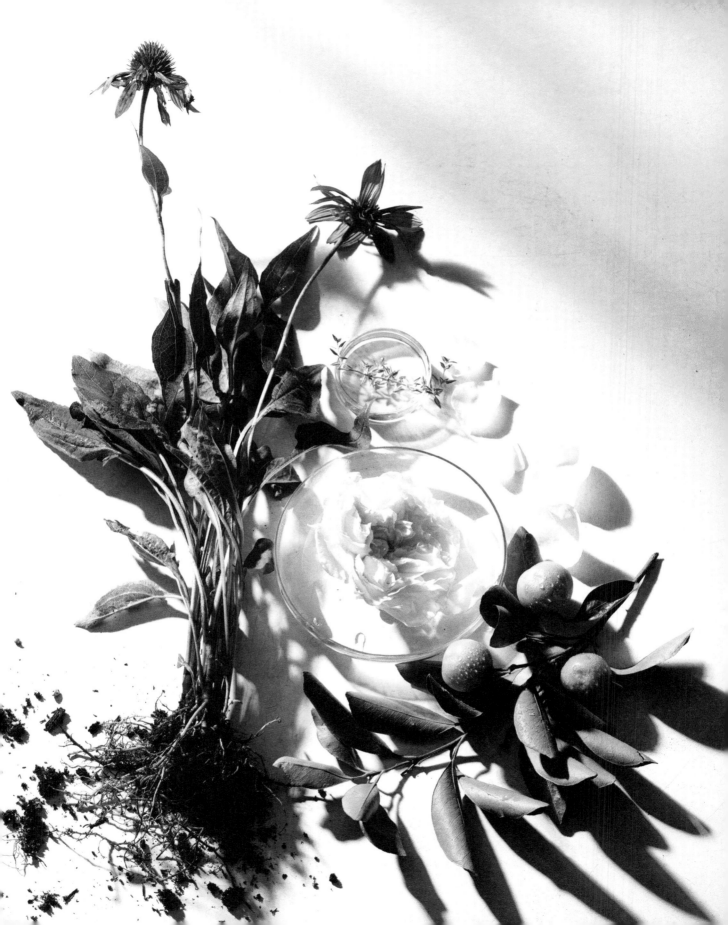

PHARMACY OF FLOWERS

Herbal medicine is the oldest and most widely used form of health care in the world. Some of the greatest healing agents have been derived from the plant kingdom and are still used throughout the world today. Many herbs have an enormous range of healing powers that can act as a restorative tonic to help the body function optimally.

Several herbs in particular are especially useful in skin care. Some herbs, such as Oregon graperoot, milk thistle, dandelion root, and burdock root, are purifying to the skin and digestive tract when taken internally, especially in detoxifying the liver, and, therefore useful for inflamed skin conditions such as acne, eczema, or psoriasis. There are other herbs that, when used externally, are helpful for their ability to calm red, irritated or inflamed skin. German chamomile, oats and aloe are all well known for their soothing properties, and calendula and gotu kola are prized for their wound-healing properties by speeding up skin barrier repair.

Herbs called adaptogens—ashwagandha, schisandra, Holy basil, and Siberian ginseng, to name a few—help to increase the body's resistance to stress. Adaptogens work by modulating the release of stress hormones from the adrenal glands, in particular cortisol, as well as epinephrine (adrenaline). By reducing the overall output of stress hormones, adaptogens help reduce anxiety, improve sleep quality, and increase mental clarity.

Nervine herbs are probably the most important group of botanicals in skin care, as they strengthen and nourish the nervous system, and calm anxiety, often a cause of many skin imbalances. Sedative herbs such as chamomile, lavender, linden blossom, skullcap, and damiana are mildly relaxing and act as general tonics to modulate stress. A stronger group of relaxing herbs called hypnotics, such as passionflower, kava root, hops, California poppy, and valerian help promote deep sleep and also work as muscle relaxants. Make sure to incorporate these herbs into the healthy sleep habits outlined on page 127.

Depending upon your skin personality, you will definitely want to keep some of these herbal remedies on hand and can purchase these herbs from a specialty herbal-remedy company (see Resources section). Herbs can be ingested as teas, as a gentle tonic, or as tinctures. Herbal tinctures, also known as liquid herbal extracts, are the original U.S. Pharmacopeia method for extracting herbs. Herbalists consider tinctures more effective than capsules or powdered herbs, as this form best preserves the active constituents, assures potency, and they assimilate into the bloodstream more quickly. Extracted in an alcohol and water base, tinctures are concentrated remedies and are taken by the dropperful several times a day either neat or added to water, juice, or tea.

Externally, herbs also can be applied to the skin as salves, oils or ointments. Allow time to make some of these preparations yourself and enjoy participating in your own healing regimen.

German chamomile, oats and aloe are all well-known for their soothing properties, and calendula and gotu kola are prized for their wound-healing properties by speeding up skin barrier repair.

HOME HERBAL-REMEDY CHEST

HERB	PROPERTIES	APPLICATIONS	INSTRUCTIONS	PRECAUTIONS
Ashwaganda *Withania somnifera*	Adaptogen, helps body adapt to stress, soothes anxiety and increases energy	Take in liquid tincture form with other nervine herbs.	In tincture form, add 40 drops twice daily to tea or water.	Avoid during pregnancy or while nursing.
Burdock Root *Articum lappa compositae*	Blood purifier, rich in iron and minerals	Take in liquid tincture form with other skin-clarifying herbs.	In tincture form, add 40 drops twice daily to tea or water.	Avoid during pregnancy or while nursing.
Calendula *Clendula officinalis*	Wound healer and skin soother	Use externally as balm.	Apply to affected areas (see Healing Calendula Balm recipe page 138).	None
Chamomile *Matricaria chamomilla*	Anti-inflammatory; Sedative to digestive and nervous system	Use externally to soothe skin. Use internally to relax nerves.	Apply to affected areas. Add 2 teaspoons fresh herb (1 teaspoon dried) to hot water and steep for 10 minutes for a soothing tea.	None when taken at recommended dosage.
Chaste Berry *Vitex agnus-Castus*	Hormone balancing herb used to support reproductive health	Use internally to ease symptoms associated with hormonal swings.	In tincture form, add 40 drops twice daily to tea or water.	Avoid during pregnancy or while nursing.
Dandelion Root *Taraxacum officinalis)*	Liver herb used to detoxify the entire system	Take in liquid tincture form with other skin-clarifying herbs.	In tincture form, add 40 drops twice daily to tea or water.	Avoid during pregnancy or while nursing.
Evening Primrose *Oenothera biennis*	Effective skin-soothing herb due to high gamma-linolenic acid content	Take in capsule form or use externally on the skin as serum.	Take 500 mg twice daily or as directed by a physician to promote healthy skin.	None at recommended dose.
Matcha Green Tea *Camellia sinensus*	High chlorophyll levels assist with detoxification	Drink powdered form called matcha as tea.	Whisk 1 teaspoon matcha powder with 2 fluid ounces of hot water (175°F) until frothy. See Moringa Matcha Latte recipe on page 144.	Light caffeine.
Milk Thistle *Silybum marianum*	Liver tonic	Take in liquid tincture form with other skin-clarifying herbs.	In tincture form, add 40 drops twice daily to tea or water.	Avoid during pregnancy or while nursing.
Oats *Avena sativa*	Anti-inflammatory; sedative to nervous system	Use externally to calm irritated skin. Use internally as nerve tonic.	Apply to affected areas. In tincture form, add 40 drops twice daily to tea or water.	None when taken at recommended dosage.

HERB	PROPERTIES	APPLICATIONS	INSTRUCTIONS	PRECAUTIONS
Oregon Grape Root *Mahonia aquifolium*	Anti-bacterial, assists in detoxification	Take in liquid tincture form with other skin-clarifying herbs.		Avoid during pregnancy or while nursing.
Passionflower	Hypnotic; Helps promote sleep	Take in liquid tincture form with other nervine herbs.	In tincture form, add 40 drops to water or tea before bedtime.	Avoid during pregnancy or while nursing.
Psyllium Husk	Aids in sluggish digestion	Take in capsule form to keep intestines clear.	Take 1000 mg with a minimum of 8 ounces of water.	Avoid during pregnancy. Drink plenty of water as directed.
Reishi	Adaptogen herb, helps body adapt to stress, especially with lowered immunity	Take in liquid form or add dried root to soups (see page 123).	In tincture form, add 40 drops to tea or water.	Avoid during pregnancy.
Schisandra	Adaptogen, helps body adapt to stress and assists in liver detoxification	Take in liquid tincture form or infused with honey along with other adaptogen herbs.	In tincture form, add 40 drops twice daily to tea or water. See Black Cherry and Cardamom recipe on page 142.	Avoid during pregnancy or while nursing.
Siberian Ginseng *Eleutherococcus senticosus*	Adaptogen, helps body adapt to stress and helps reduce fatigue	Take in liquid tincture form or infused with honey along with other adaptogen herbs.	In tincture form, add 40 drops twice daily to tea or water. In fortified honey, add to tea.	Avoid during pregnancy or while nursing.
Skullcap *Scutellaria lateriflora*	Sedative to nervous system	Take in liquid tincture form with other relaxing herbs.	In tincture form, add 40 drops twice daily to tea or water.	Avoid during pregnancy or while nursing.
Turmeric *Curcuma longa*	Anti-inflammatory; helps to support gut health	Take in liquid tincture form with other anti-inflammatory herbs.	In tincture form, add 40 drops twice daily to tea or water. Sprinkle on food as condiment or try the Golden Turmeric Latte recipe on page 109.	Avoid during pregnancy or while nursing.
Valerian	Sedative	Take in liquid tincture form with other relaxing herbs to promote sleep.	In tincture form, add 40 drops twice daily to tea or water.	Avoid during pregnancy or while nursing.
Yellow Dock	Liver tonic and clarifying herb for the skin	Take in liquid tincture form with other skin-clarifying herbs.	In tincture form, add 40 drops twice daily to tea or water.	Avoid during pregnancy or while nursing.

HERBAL PRESCRIPTIONS

The following recipes provide solutions to everyday skin care complaints. Use them to supplement your personalized beauty regimen.

Healing Calendula Balm

MAKES	½ ounce
PREP TIME	30 minutes
YOU WILL NEED	one ½-ounce dark-colored glass ointment jar

A HR SR M

This all-natural version of "bag balm," a well-known farmer's salve, is perfect for dry, irritated, or chapped skin. Calendula is traditionally known as a wound-healer and its anti-inflammatory properties make it excellent for eczema, psoriasis, acute dermatitis, or a wound or burn. The beeswax base is quickly absorbed into the skin, leaving your skin smooth and soft without the greasy feel that petrochemical bases such as mineral oil or paraffin leave behind.

½ ounce Calendula Oil (page 69)

½ tablespoon grated beeswax

3 drops rose *(Rosa damascena)* essential oil

2 drops neroli *(Citrus aurantium)* essential oil

Pour the calendula oil and beeswax into a heatproof glass measuring cup. Place the cup in a shallow pan of simmering water. Heat, stirring constantly, until the ingredients are melted together. Remove from the heat, add the rose and neroli essential oils, and stir until well mixed. Pour into the ointment jar and place in the refrigerator to set. Apply liberally to your body as needed.

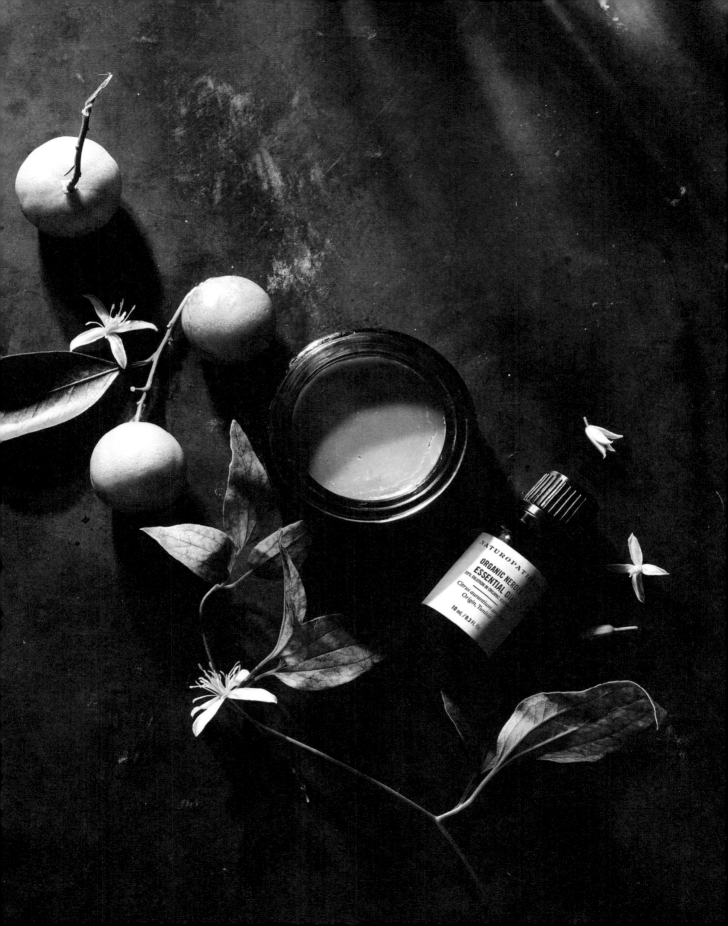

NATUROPATHI
ORGANIC NEROLI
ESSENTIAL OIL
10% SOLUTION IN ORGANIC JOJOBA
Citrus aurantium amara
Origin: Tunisia

10 mL / 0.3 FL OZ

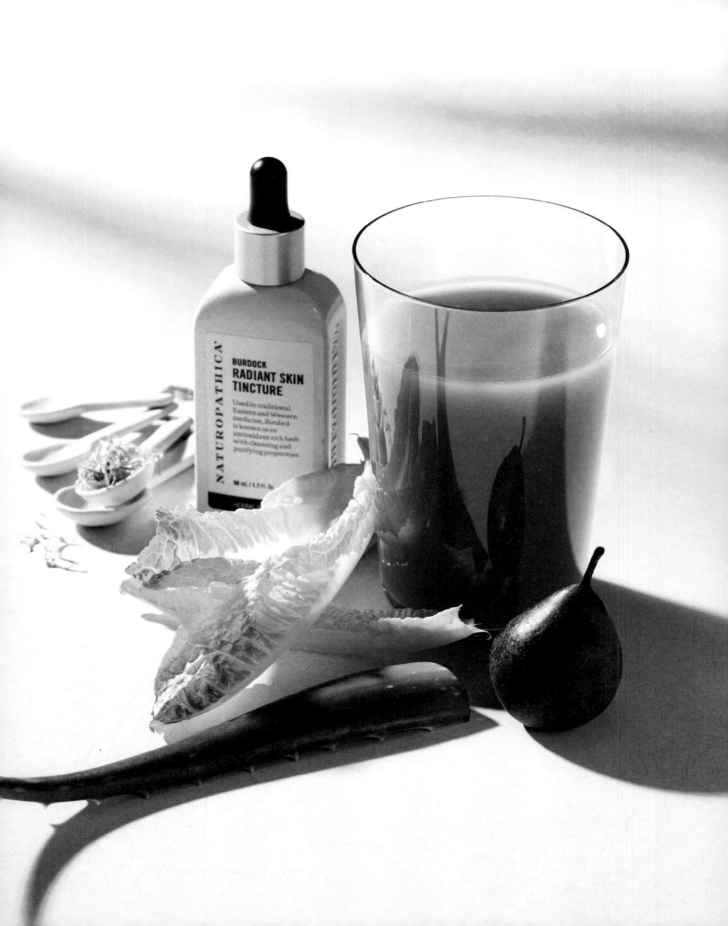

Radiant Skin Tonic

This Radiant Skin Tonic is one of the most popular green drinks at our Vitality Bar and is served with every facial treatment for its alkalizing properties to support healthy skin, hair and nails. While berries usually get the most credit when it comes to supplying antioxidants, apples are a close second. Phytonutrients such as quercetin in apples can help regulate blood sugar, useful for hormone reactive skin. In addition, apples and pears are an excellent source of dietary fiber and, when combined with healing aloe, help support a healthy gut biome.

MAKES	12 ounces
PREP TIME	15 minutes

A	HR	SR	M

TIMESAVER TIP
Try the **Naturopathica Skin Tea** or our **Burdock Radiant Skin Tincture,** which use these, along with other soothing herbs, to fortify the skin.

2 Macintosh apples

2 Anjou pears

6 ounces Skin Tea (see recipe page 145)

1 head romaine lettuce

1 cup spinach

1 medium cucumber

2 tablespoons lemon juice

2 tablespoons aloe gel

Burdock Tincture

Feed apples, pears, romaine, spinach and cucumber into a juicer—alternating the greens with the fruit. Squeeze the lemon juice into the blend and stir in the aloe vera juice.

Rosemary-Lemon Beauty Tonic

All of the guests at our healing arts centers are offered a glass of rosemary-lemon water after their session. Lemon is bursting with antioxidants like vitamin C to fight off free radicals, and rosemary is rich in two powerful antioxidants, carnosol and carnosic acid, both of which have strong anti-inflammatory properties. This tonic is highly alkalizing and can be served either warm or chilled. Sip throughout the day to promote a more vibrant complexion.

MAKES	8 ounces
PREP TIME	5 minutes

A	HR	SR	M

1 cup purified water

2 tablespoons fresh lemon juice

1 sprig fresh rosemary, crushed

Bring the water to a boil in a small saucepan. Combine the rosemary and lemon juice in a cup. Pour in the boiling water and let steep for 10 minutes. Strain and enjoy.

Black Cherry and Cardamom Shrub

MAKES	3 cups
PREP TIME	45 minutes

A HR SR M

If you have never sipped a shrub—a concoction of fruit, aromatics, honey, and vinegar that was popular in seventeenth and eighteenth century England, you are in for a real treat. Not only is this a delightfully delicious drink, but this fermented beverage is good for gut health because apple cider vinegar is rich in digestive enzymes. Shrubs are a better option than kombucha for people with candida or those who are sensitive to caffeine. In this recipe, dark-pigmented black cherries, brimming with antioxidants, are infused with schisandra, a tart berry native to China and Russia and prized as an adaptogen herb to reduce physical and mental stress. Add this zingy fruit syrup to seltzer water or add a shot of your favorite liquor to make a delicious cocktail.

1 pound black cherries

1 tablespoon whole cardamom pods

2 tablespoons schisandra berries

1 cinnamon stick

2 cups honey

1 cup apple cider vinegar, or to taste

Using a paring knife, slice up the cherries into a bowl, removing the pits if needed. Squeeze with your hand to release the juices. Gently crush cardamom pods in a mortar using a pestle and add to the mixture. Add the schisandra berries and cinnamon stick and then pour the honey over the mixture and stir to mix well. Let the mixture sit, covered with a clean dish towel on the countertop, for about 2 days, stirring once a day to combine the juices.

Strain the mixture into a measuring cup, discarding the solids. Slowly add the apple cider vinegar, sampling the shrub periodically until you get the acidity that you like. Transfer to a jar and cover tightly with the lid. Store in the refrigerator for up to 3 months.

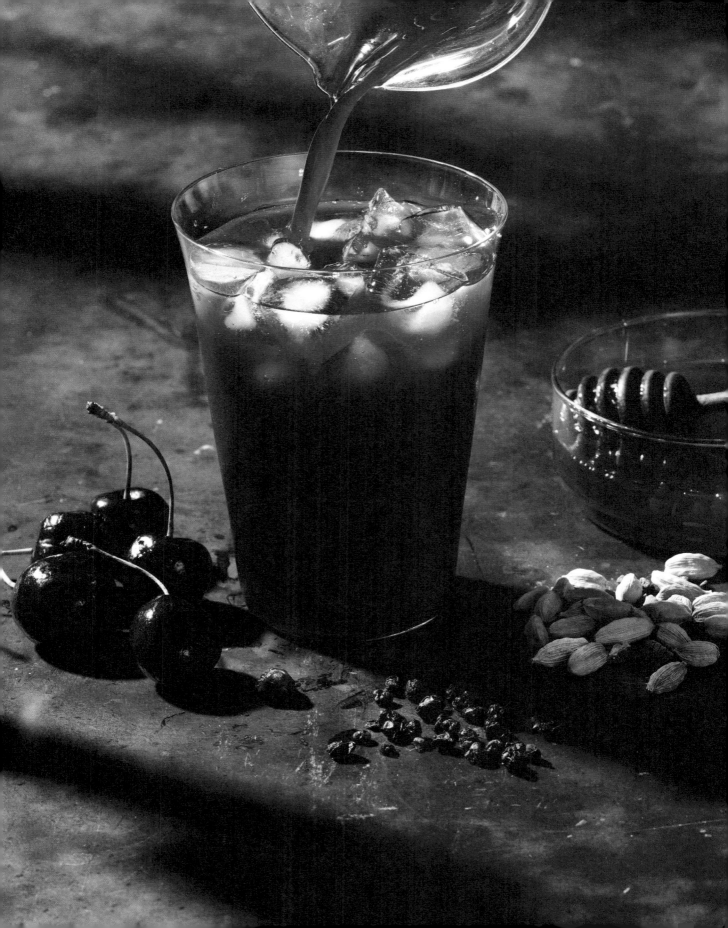

Moringa Matcha Latte

MAKES	1 serving
PREP TIME	10 minutes

A HR SR M

On days when I cannot find the time to make a green juice or smoothie, I turn to this delicious beverage, which is easy to prepare. One of my favorite herbs, moringa, is super-rich in antioxidants to fight cellular damage that ages the skin. Animal studies suggest that moringa provides analgesic and anti-inflammatory properties.[4] Here, it is paired with matcha, a finely ground powder of premium green tea that is a powerhouse: one serving of matcha tea has 2 to 3 times the antioxidants, called epigallocatechin gallate, or EGCG, of regular sencha green tea. Some people refer to matcha as liquid chlorophyll, since unlike other green teas, matcha is not processed, so it delivers more nutrients. In addition, matcha is rich in the amino acid theanine, which studies have shown induces a relaxed but alert mental state.

¾ cup unsweetened almond milk, preferably homemade (page 115)

½ teaspoon moringa powder

½ teaspoon matcha powder

1 tablespoon hot water

Maple syrup or stevia

In a saucepan, heat the almond milk to just simmering. Remove from the heat and pour into a heatproof ceramic bowl. Using a whisk or immersion blender, froth the milk. Set aside.

Combine the moringa and matcha powders in a separate bowl and add the hot water. Whisk with a bamboo or metal whisk until completely dissolved. Sweeten with the maple syrup or stevia to taste. Pour into a cup and top off with the steamed milk. Drink hot.

Golden Turmeric Latte

Brightly colored turmeric has long been used to support a healthy inflammatory response in the body. Traditionally, it is paired with ginger to support digestive health along with black pepper and fat-soluble coconut milk so that the active component in turmeric, curcumin, can pass through the small intestine and absorb into the bloodstream. Here it is paired with cinnamon bark to help maintain normal blood sugar, making it a useful staple for Hormone Reactive skin (see page 23), as well as the adaptogen herb ashwagandha to build energy reserves and stamina.

MAKES	2 servings
PREP TIME	10 minutes

A HR SR M

1 cup unsweetened almond milk, preferably homemade (page 115)

1 cup coconut milk

1½ teaspoons ground turmeric, plus more for serving

¼ teaspoon ashwagandha

¼ teaspoon ground ginger

¼ teaspoon whole cardamom pods

1 cinnamon stick

Pinch of freshly ground black pepper

1 tablespoon unrefined virgin coconut oil

1 tablespoon maple syrup, honey, or stevia

In a saucepan, combine the almond milk, coconut milk, turmeric, ashwagandha, ginger, cardamom pods, cinnamon stick, black pepper, coconut oil, and maple syrup over medium heat until simmering. Cover, reduce heat, and simmer for 5 minutes.

Remove from the heat; strain and discard the solids. Whisk or use an immersion blender until frothy. Divide between two cups and sprinkle with more ground turmeric. Serve hot.

Skin Tea

This elegant tea is excellent for all Skin Personalities (see pages 30–46). Soothing, lush blossoms of healing calendula and red clover, a traditional blood-cleansing herb, are entwined with calming lemon balm and nestled in a bed of antioxidant-rich green tea. Serve hot or chilled.

MAKES	2 cups
PREP TIME	5 minutes

A HR SR M

TIMESAVER TIP
Try the **Naturopathica Skin Tea,** which uses these herbs as well as other soothing extracts to fortify the skin.

1 teaspoon green tea

¼ cup fresh red clover blossoms or ⅛ cup dried

2 teaspoons fresh calendula blossoms or 1 teaspoon dried

2 teaspoons fresh lemon balm or 1 teaspoon dried

2 teaspoons fresh lavender or 1 teaspoon dried

2 cups purified water (1½ if making iced tea)

Combine all the herbal ingredients in a French press. Pour in boiling water and let the tea steep for 10 minutes. For acute skin conditions such as eczema or dermatitis, drink 4 cups a day until symptoms abate.

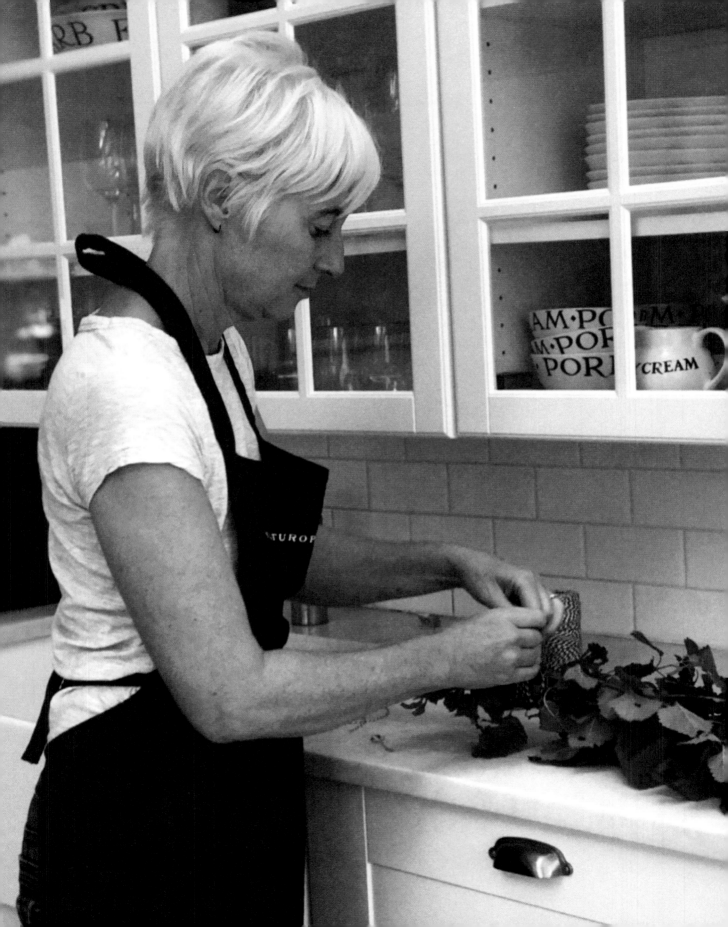

Herbal Tinctures

Herbal tinctures are liquid extracts of herbs. They are prepared by combining a fresh or dried herb in a solvent, usually an alcohol and water, or glycerin base, resulting in a higher concentration of the active herbal ingredient than you would find in an herbal tea.

The tincture preparation below is known as the "folk method" because it requires only basic measuring and is good for general use for the home herbal remedy chest. Professionally prepared tinctures calculate the exact weight of the herb and the volume of the solvent or menstruum in order to provide a specific tincture strength and more exact dosage.

Dried herb of your choice **80-proof or 100-proof vodka**

Using a coffee grinder, or in a mortar using a pestle, grind your dried herb into a coarse powder. Place the powder in the canning jar. Add the vodka until it covers the herb, stir to mix well, and then add an additional ¼ inch of vodka on top of the herb (if the herb is floating, make sure there is ¼ inch of vodka below it). Cap tightly and set aside in a cool place, away from direct sunlight.

Check the following day and if the herb has absorbed all the vodka, add more to re-establish ¼ inch of extra liquid. Shake the tincture daily for 14 days. Pour the liquid into a measuring cup through a strainer or coffee filter, pressing on the pulp to release as much tincture as possible. Pour the tincture into the bottles, cap tightly, and label with the name of tincture and date prepared.

MAKES	Approximately 1 quart
PREP TIME	20 minutes
YOU WILL NEED	1-ounce dark-colored glass bottles, as many as you need to hold the amount of tincture you make; one 1-quart canning jar

A   HR   SR   M

Stress Tea

This recipe contains two sedative herbs, chamomile and passionflower, along with two adaptogens, holy basil and schisandra, to modulate stress hormones. Make this tea one hour before bedtime and then nestle under the covers with a good book. If you are lucky, you will remember to turn off the light before drifting off to sleep.

1 cup purified water

¼ teaspoon dried chamomile flowers

¼ teaspoon dried lavender flowers

¼ teaspoon dried holy basil

¼ teaspoon dried schisandra berry

30 to 40 drops passionflower tincture

Bring the water to a boil in a small saucepan. Put the herbs in a heatproof bowl and pour in the boiling water. Let steep for 10 minutes. Strain into a cup and add the passionflower tincture. Stir and enjoy.

MAKES	1 cup
PREP TIME	10 minutes

A   HR   SR   M

TIMESAVER TIP
Try the **Naturopathica Stress Tea,** which uses all of these herbs as well as other soothing extracts to fortify the skin.

BEAUTY DOPP KIT

During World War II, recruits were issued travel kits, called "Dopp kits," that contained all standard-issue and emergency gear that a soldier carried on a regular basis.

In order to achieve healthy skin that focuses on beauty from within and not just topical treatments, you will need to stock up on the essentials listed below to create your own beauty Dopp kit. Make this your go-to for all of your holistic skin care needs.

The Green Routine

Open your medicine cabinet and check the labels of your skin care products. If any contain some of the ingredients listed on pages 51–52, toss them in the waste bin. Purchase skin-friendly, clean beauty-care essentials: sulfate-free cleanser, exfoliant, toner, facial oil, moisturizer, eye cream, and sunblock. These basics will go a long way towards helping you look your best.

Herbal Remedies

Herbs contain many highly active ingredients and balancing secondary ingredients that work synergistically to make them a potent form of natural medicine. Herbal medicines work in a variety of ways to assist skin metabolism. Herbs support healthy digestion by acting as "prebiotics" through providing food for the good bacteria in your gut to flourish which in turn benefits the skin. Herbs called adaptogens help increase your body's resistance to stress and disease by boosting immunity and modulating cortisol which protects us from burn out.

The following skin-clarifying herbs are potent allies in helping the skin function optimally through their ability to detoxify the body, calm inflammation or by helping your body adapt to stress: dandelion root, milk thistle, yellow dock, oregon grape root, burdock root, calendula, stinging nettle, green tea extract, ashwagandha, schisandra, and holy basil. Taken alone or combined, these herbs can be ingested as a liquid extract or in capsule form.

Herbs support healthy digestion by acting as "prebiotics" through providing food for the good bacteria in your gut to flourish, which in turn benefits the skin.

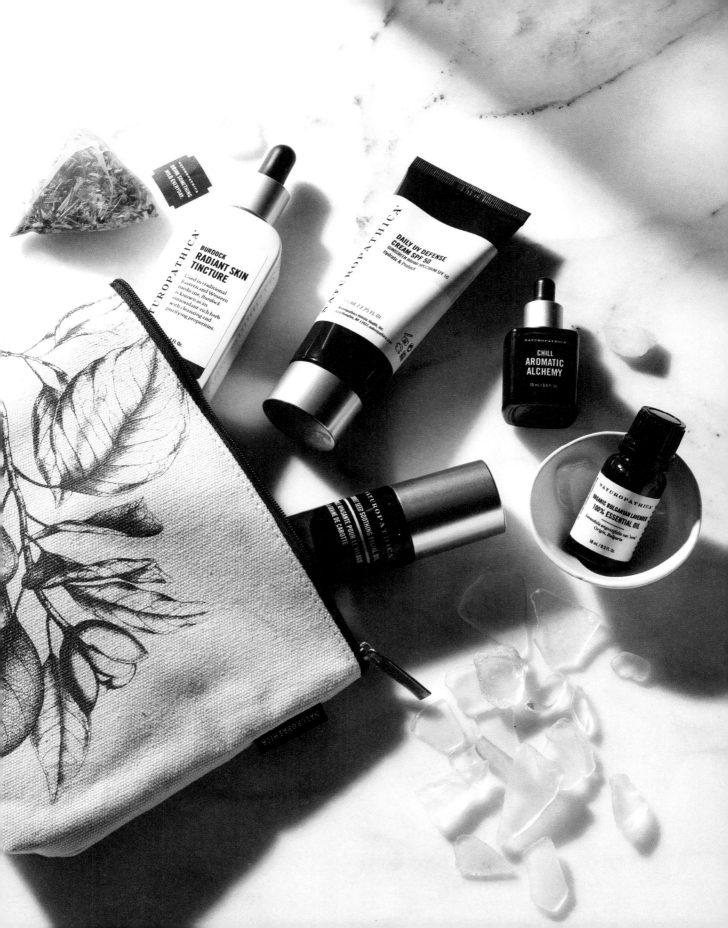

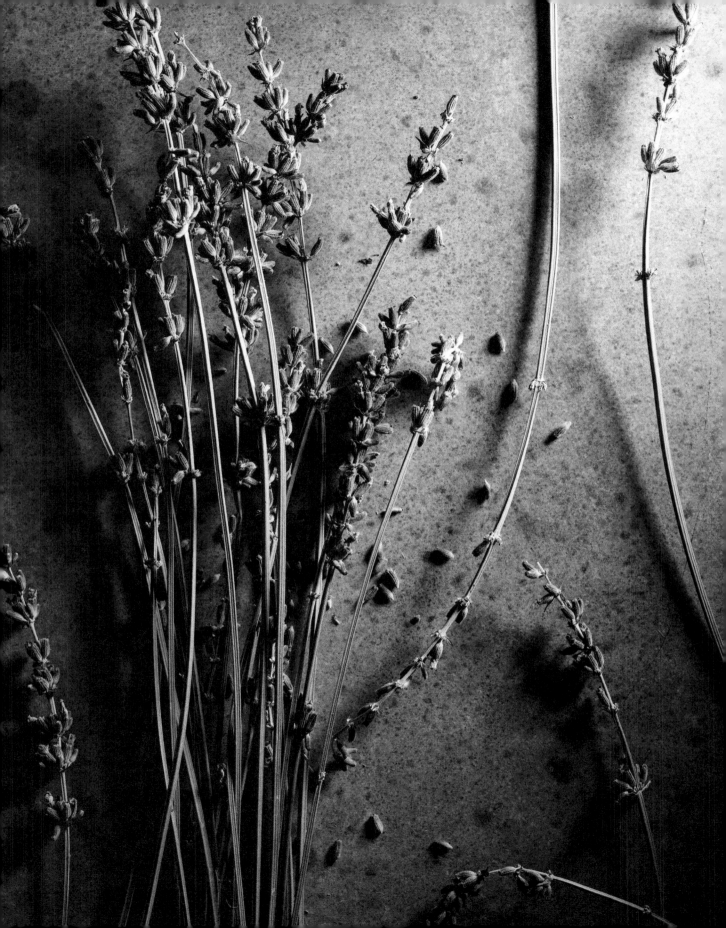

BEAUTY DOPP KIT *(Continued)*

Beauty Vitamins and Supplements

Good health comes from good food. However, special supplements like essential fatty acids or probiotics or a good multivitamin go a long way towards ensuring that your skin has what it needs. Vitamin A is essential for normal development of skin and other epithelial tissues, B-complex vitamins helps bring blood to the tissues, and Vitamin C is essential for its role as a powerful antioxidant. Many people are deficient in Vitamin D3 due to lack of exposure to sunlight. Vitamin D3 helps to manage skin conditions like rosacea and eczema, so be sure to supplement if your skin is sensitive.

If you are time-compressed or traveling, drink Vitamin Water or add an effervescent vitamin packet to water or juice.

Flower Essences

During the 1930s, Dr Edward Bach discovered the 38 Flower Essences. These homeopathically prepared remedies represent a complete system of healing directed at personality, mood, and the emotional outlook of an individual.

Since stress is at the root of many skin imbalances, make sure to include flower essences in your Beauty Dopp kit to soothe emotional upsets. Include Bach's Rescue Remedy or try a custom blend of remedies that would work best for your particular needs.

Aromatherapy

Aromatherapy is the art and science of using the volatile essential oils of plants—often referred to as a plant's "life force"—for healing. Genuine essential oils—not synthetic fragrances—can assist in the maintenance of healthy skin from treating blemishes and rashes to keeping your moods balanced.

Keep lavender oil in your Dopp kit, a useful first aid to help keep stress at bay, as well as tea tree oil to treat breakouts and blemishes. Place 3 drops of Mandarin oil on a tissue and put under your pillowcase to help you sleep.

ASSORTED ESSENTIALS

These are the extras you can't live without:

- ☐ **Natural Baby Wipes** These are great for removing heavy oil-based make up.

- ☐ **Sleep Mask** A comfortable eye mask is essential beauty sleep.

- ☐ **Healing Balm** A good beeswax balm is essential for relieving dry patches of skin, healing cuticles, sealing in extra moisture on the face, or even styling the hair.

- ☐ **Carrot Seed Oil** Rich in Omega-3 and Omega-6 fatty acids to calm down inflammation, this oil leaves a matte finish and penetrates the deepest layers of the epidermis.

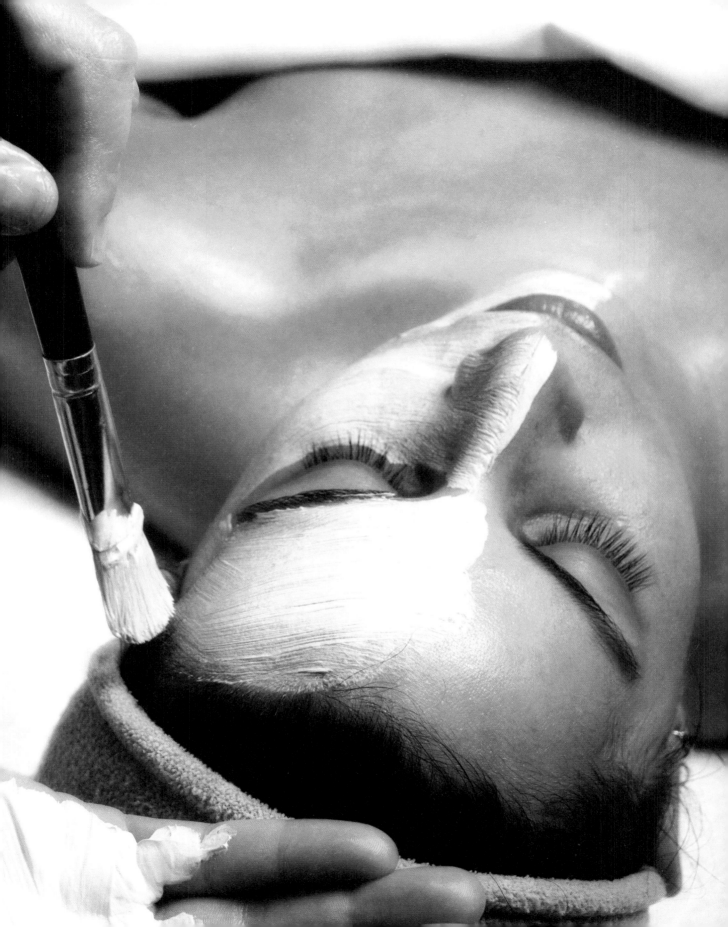

Resources

American Association of Naturopathic Physicians (AANP)
A recommended resource for finding qualified naturopathic doctors and natural-health publications and information.
http://www.naturopathic.org

818 18th St. NW, Suite 250
Washington, DC 20006
(866) 538-2267

American Herbalists Guild
A good resource for finding qualified herbalists and information about best practices for herbal medicine.
www.americanherbalistsguild.com

P.O. Box 3076
Asheville, NC 28802-3076
(617) 520-4372

Mountain Rose Herbs
A favorite resource for high-quality herbs, spices, beeswax, carrier oils, and natural base creams.
www.mountainroseherbs.com

P.O. Box 50220
Eugene, OR 97405
(800) 879-3337

Naturopathica
Naturopathica pairs natural ingredients with clean actives to create skin care, body care, and herbal remedies that deliver true and lasting results. Shop our website for our full range of products along with wellness resources and a list of our Spa Partners to help you look and feel your best from the inside out.
Naturopathica.com

Naturopathica Healing Arts Center & Spa—East Hampton
At Naturopathica East Hampton, we've been inspiring our community to re-boot, relax, and live well for over twenty years. Our passion for wellness translates into holistic facials and herbal massages using our celebrated skin and body products.

74 Montauk Hwy
East Hampton, NY 11937
(631) 329-2525

Naturopathica Healing Arts Center & Spa—Chelsea
Our flagship spa in New York City brings the Naturopathica experience to life. Through our signature holistic facials and herbal massages, Sensory & Meditation Lounge, classes, Vitality Bar of Herbal Remedies, and award-winning product selection, Naturopathica Chelsea offers holistic solutions that provide true and lasting results.

127 W. 26th Street
New York, NY 10001
(646) 979-3960

SKS Bottle & Packaging
www.sks-bottle.com

2600 7th Avenue
Watervliet, NY 12189
(518) 880-6980 Ext. 1

References

CHAPTER 1

[1] Digestive Disease Statistics for the United States, National Institute of Diabetes and Digestive and Kidney Disease, National Institute of Health https://www.niddk.nih.gov/health-information/health-statistics/digestive-diseases

[2] Bischoff, S., Barbara, G., Buurman, W., Ockhulzen, T., Schulzke, J., Serino, M,, Tilg, H., Watson, A., and Wells, J. (2014). *Intestinal permeability— a new target for disease prevention and therapy.* BMC Gastroenterology, November 14: 189.

CHAPTER 2

[1] Talbott, W. and Duffy, N. (2015). *Complementary and alternative medicine for psoriasis: what the dermatologist needs to know.* American Journal of Clinical Dermatology, June; 16(3): 147-65.

CHAPTER 3

[1] Ecovia Intelligence, Sustainable Cosmetics Summit, May 2017.

[2] Mintel Market Research, *Sensitive Skin Claims Represent a Quarter of New US Launches in 2014.* http://www.mintel.com/press-centre/beauty-and-personal-care/us-facial-skincare-trends

CHAPTER 4

[1] Murray, C., Ng, Marie., and Mokdad, A. (2014). The vast majority of American adults are overweight or obese, and weight is a growing problem among US children. Institute for Health Metrics and Evaluation, http://www.healthdata.org

[2] Davis, D. (2009). *Declining fruit and vegetable nutrient composition: what is the evidence?* HortScience, February; 44(1): 15-19.

[3] Bechthold, A., Boeing, H., Schwed-helm, C., Hoffmann, G., Knuppel, S., Iqbal, K..... and Schwingshackl, L. (2017). *Food groups and risk of coronary heart disease, stroke and heart failure: a systematic review and dose-response meta-analysis of prospective studies.* Clinical Reviews in Food Science and Nutrition, October; 17:0.

[4] Foster, J., Rinaman, L. and Cryan, J. (2017). *Stress and the gut-brain axis.* Neurobiology of Stress, December; 7: 124-136.

CHAPTER 5

[1] Nerurkar, A., Bitton, A., Davis, R., Phillips, R. and Yeh, G. (2013). *When physicians counsel about stress: results of a national study.* Journal of the American Medical Association, January; 14; 173(1): 76-77.

[2] Center for Disease Control and Prevention, National Center for Health Statistics. *Antidepressant Use in Persons Aged 12 and Over: United States, 2005-2008 (2011).* NCHS Data Brief, October; 76.

[3] Duraimani, S., Schneider, R., Randall, O., Nidich, S., Xu, S., Ketete, M.... and Fagan, J. (2015). *Effects of lifestyle modification on telomerase gene expression in hypertensive patients: a pilot trial of stress reduction and health education programs in African Americans.* PLOS ONE, November 16, https://doi.org/10.1371/journal.pone.0142689

[4] Tamrat, Y., Nedi, T., Assefa, S., Teklehaymanot, T., Shibeshi, W. (2017). *Anti-inflammatory and analgesic activities of solvent fractions of the leaves of Moringa stenopetala bak. (Moringaceae) in mice models.* BioMed Central Complementary Alternative Medicine, September 29; 17(1): 473.

Index

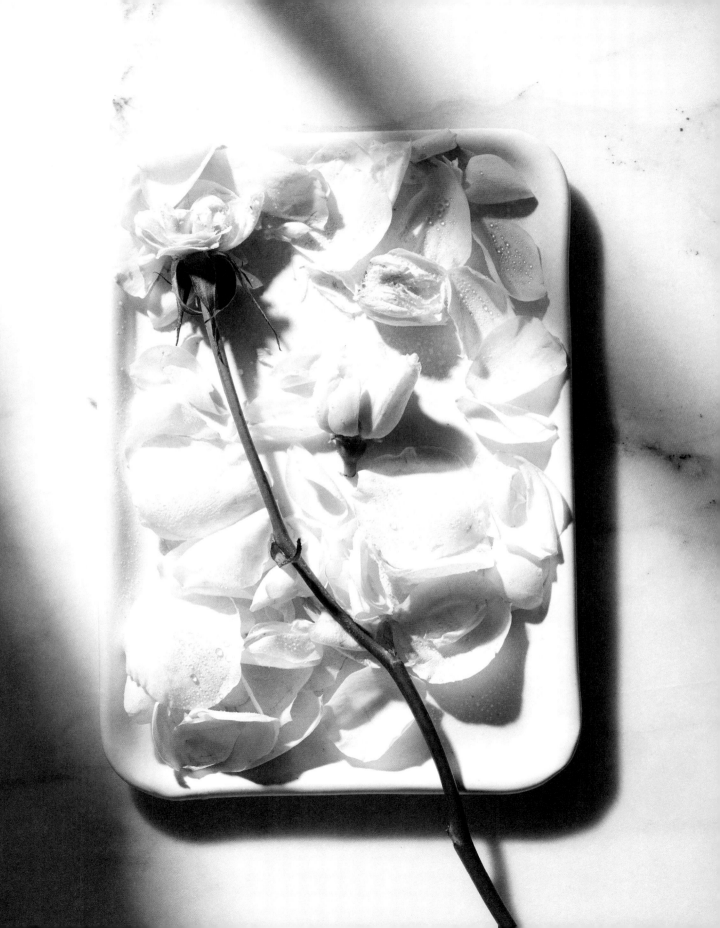

Photograph on p. 8 by Catherine
Chermayeff; photograph on pp. 12–13
by Kevin Gilgan/Stocksy United;
photograph on p. 14 by Andrei Aleshyn/
Stocksy United; photograph on p. 35
by Susan Brooks-Dammann/Stocksy
United; photograph on p. 57 and p. 96
by Anna Williams; photograph on p. 63
by Nadine Greeff/Stocksy United;
photograph on p. 85 by Lumina/Stocksy
United; photograph on p. 86 by
Catherine Chermayeff; photograph on
p. 93 by Pixel Stories/Stocksy United;
photograph on p. 106 by Tatjana
Zlatkovic/Stocksy United; photograph
on pp. 124–125 by Michela Ravasio/
Stocksy United; photograph on p. 131
by Martin Benik/Westend61/Offset.com;
photograph on p. 146 by Catherine
Chermayeff; photograph on p. 150 by
David De Stefano/Offset.com; photograph on p. 152 by YanC/iStock.com

All other photographs by Kate Mathis.

ISBN 9781388853433
First Publishing, 2005,
Pure Skin: Organic Beauty Basics

Manufactured in China

Design by Alisha Petro

FDA DISCLAIMER
These herbal remedies have not been
evaluated by the Food and Drug
Administration and are not intended
to diagnose, cure, mitigate, treat, or
prevent disease. The author is not
responsible for any effects or conse-
quences that may result from the use
of these remedies. The remedies are
created from traditional sources of
herbal knowledge.

Acknowledgments

I am grateful to all of the wonderful
people who helped *The Naturopathica
Effect: A Holistic Approach to Skin Care*
come into being. First and foremost,
to all the herbalists who have passed
down the ancestral knowledge of herbal
medicine and the therapeutic properties
of plants. Without their unwavering
commitment to ensuring that herbal
medicine is an accessible and valuable
part of health care, this book would not
be possible. Thanks also to the whole
team at Naturopathica, especially
Emily, for her editing expertise, and
Eon, for her design input. A special
thanks to Kate Mathis, for her beautiful
photography, and Pamela Duncan Silver,
for her amazing styling. Thanks to
Stefanie Sacks and Talia Segal Fidler,
whose nutritional consulting helped
guide several recipes of this book.
A special thanks to Carrie Bradley
Neves, who assisted with copyediting
and was instrumental in helping guide
me through this process. And lastly,
thanks to my husband, Courtney, who
adds so much joy to my life and whose
patience created the space for me to
write this book.